How to

Stress, Depression, and Anxiety

A Vital Guide on How to Deal with Nerves and Coping with Stress, Pain, OCD and Trauma

Richard Banks

Thank You!

Thank you for your purchase.

I am dedicated to making the most enriching and informational content. I hope it meets your expectations and you gain a lot from it.

Your comments and feedback are important to me because they help me to provide the best material possible. So, if you have any questions or concerns, please email me at richardbanks.books@gmail.com.

Again, thank you for your purchase.

INTRODUCTION

Congratulations on purchasing *How to Deal with Stress, Depression, and Anxiety,* and thank you for doing so.

Virtually all people experience stress, anxiety, or depression at various points in their lives. One 2017 study suggested that about 792 million people worldwide have formal mental health disorders, with depression and anxiety being the most common conditions. Millions, maybe even billions, of additional people experience subclinical conditions and high levels of stress, so the number of people who deal daily with such issues is quite astounding. When you live with any of these conditions, everyday activities become a challenge, and you may resort to self-sabotaging behaviors, or you feel stuck in place.

As these conditions continue, it only makes you feel worse, both mentally and physically. In the United States, it's been reported that stress affects the mental health of 73 percent of the population, leading to worsening conditions like depression and anxiety. While these conditions are all too common, they don't have to be. Living with mental illness or stress can feel impossible, and that's a hard burden to carry, which is why mental distress often leads to further mental and emotional anguish.

The Challenge

With so much external pressure in today's society to be their best selves, millions of people worldwide struggle to maintain their mental health and professional or personal well-being.

Many emotionally and physically harmful behaviors—such as overworking and extreme self-sacrifice—are glorified by society. As people are pushed to do their best work and make room for a personal and social life, they can become consumed by anxiety and worries that impede their progress.

The statistics on stress, anxiety, and depression depict a grim picture. As the most prevalent mental health issue in the United States, according to the Anxiety and Depression Association of America, anxiety impacts over 40 million American adults, representing over 18 percent of the population. Globally, nearly 300 million people have anxiety. People who have anxiety tend to have greater stress levels, and 50 percent of those diagnosed with anxiety will also be diagnosed with depression. Depression rates are also startlingly high, with just under seven percent of the population experiencing major depression at any given time and another two percent experiencing persistent depressive disorder, also known as dysthymia or chronic depression.

Even if you don't have a clinically diagnosed issue, such as depression or anxiety, you likely have some degree of stress that makes it harder to function as you'd like to. The Global Organization for Stress says that 75 percent of people are moderately stressed, and nearly all people experience stress at some point in their lives because of a myriad of contributing factors. With so much mental dysfunction, it's no wonder that some people think they'll never get better, but this grim picture doesn't have to be your reality.

While mental health conditions have the power to destroy and debilitate people—paralyzing them and making it hard to have hope for the future— there are proven techniques anyone can use to improve their mental health and allow greater opportunity for personal development. You do not

10

need to let your stress, anxiety, or depression hold you back anymore.

The solution to managing your mental health isn't easy or quick, but it is effective. With effort and careful attention to a multi-faceted plan, you can make dramatic improvements to your damaged mental health and start investing more energy into things that make you the most gratified. There are several steps you must follow for the best results. When you apply these steps, you can have increased mental clarity, emotional freedom, and confidence. Curing your mental health issues will require you to face everything that scares you and to admit uncomfortable truths. Still, you'll be far better off when you seek help than the nearly 25 million Americans who have untreated mental health conditions. You may not need the same level of care as people with more severe conditions, but you do need help because living with any degree of stress, anxiety, or depression is living with more pain than you need to have.

Treating a mental illness can seem intimidating to many people, but there are several effective methods, and there are ways to treat, if not cure, any mental health condition you may have. With so many adults and children not currently being treated for their mental health issues, it's no wonder that mental health statistics remain so prevalent. Still, with increased awareness and the greater availability of mental health resources, the prognosis for those who have mental illness continues to improve. Alongside this, as these issues become more widely acknowledged and discussed, the stigmas attached to them are beginning to dissipate, which removes some of the shame linked to mental illness, which only exacerbates it. Accordingly, by committing bravely to treatment and opening yourself to increased understanding of mental illness, you create resilience against mental illness and become more proactive in the treatment of these debilitating conditions.

For those of you with any of these issues, you cannot delay treatment. Mental dysfunction of any kind makes it harder to feel joy and, in the worst cases, it can deprive you of your ability to function. More than that, your mental health can also impact your physical health. For example, research has shown that stress increases the chance of someone dying from cancer by 32 percent. The Canadian Mental Health Association says that people with poor mental health are more prone to having chronic physical disorders.

A study from Johns Hopkins University found that patients with a family history of heart disease were healthier when they engaged in positive thinking. Among the participants of the study, those who had a positive outlook were 13 percent less likely to experience a cardiac event. Additionally, they found that, generally, people who have better outlooks live longer.

The Solution

Recovery is a process that isn't always linear, but this book will lay out the basic steps to help get you on the right track. The first step in the process is all about education. Before you can do anything else, you must understand the beast you're trying to slaughter and the sword you'll use to slay it. You'll learn how the brain works and how problems with its wiring can lead to mental dysfunction. You'll also learn how you can rewire your cognitive processes to promote increased mental health.

In the second step of the process, you'll continue your educational journey and gain a more in-depth understanding of what anxiety, stress, and depression are and how they impact the way you function. You'll start to understand how to address each of these issues using essential coping tools.

Once you've learned about each condition, you'll

be introduced to one of the most powerful psychological tools for improved mental health: Cognitive Behavioral Therapy (CBT). You'll discover what CBT is and how to use it to address your mental ailments.

Once you understand the founding principles of these conditions and the fundamentals of CBT, you'll learn how to manage your circumstances daily by overcoming roadblocks and reviving your sense of self by shifting your perspective as you begin to think in new ways. You'll start to care for both your body and your mind in life-changing ways. All of these steps will lead to mental clarity and mental liberation.

With all this in mind, it's clear that a person's mental health impacts every part of their life, and without addressing your mental dysfunction, you'll never have the peace of mind you crave. Each day you do nothing about your mental health is another day you deprive yourself of health and happiness. Your mental health should be your priority, because you cannot fully function as a member of society if you're prohibited from doing all the things you love the most.

If you feel like you are losing sight of yourself and your desires because of your stress, anxiety, or depression, it's time to make a change. It's okay to be nervous about the adjustments you will need to make to feel healthier, but remember that being uncomfortable and uncertain is vital because they represent change. If you don't change, you'll never feel better than you do now. Maybe you have learned to live with your pain and worry, but it's time to learn to live without those negative coping mechanisms because they stop you from living your life to the fullest.

While the techniques in this book can help you improve your levels of stress, anxiety, and depression, I recommend seeking professional support to help push you towards your goals

There are tons of books on this subject on the market, so thank you for choosing this one! "How to Deal with Stress, Depression, and Anxiety" will provide a complete framework and a well-rounded set of tools for you to understand the causes of stress, depression, anxiety and how to overcome it. Please enjoy!

Chapter 1: How Your Brain Works

Too many people hurt their recovery journey by working against their minds. They think they can force their brains into submission, and when that doesn't work, they feel like failures. When a change you're trying to make doesn't stick, it is usually because it isn't one your brain is used to. As much as you may want that change, your brain will resist it because unfamiliar things feel unsafe to the human brain. The human brain loves patterns, and it uses those patterns to create your internal mental programming and perceptions of reality. When you understand how your brain works, you can use it to your advantage to create new patterns and reframe your mental state.

Your brain is a powerful force, and it can work in remarkable ways. In facing your worries, doubts, and other negative feelings, you need to understand how your brain functions so you can stop fighting your brain and start working with it.

Your Map of Reality

In 1931, scientist and philosopher Alfred Korzybski established an important metaphorical notion with his statement, "The map is not the territory." He believed that individuals don't have absolute knowledge of reality; instead, they have a set of beliefs built up over time that influence how they perceive events and situations. People's beliefs and views (their map) are not reality itself (the territory). In other words, perception is not reality.

Your brain fills gaps in understanding automatically. This means that when you don't know something, you subconsciously make an estimation based on the information you do know. When you experience worry or sadness, this can be caused by a map of reality that reinforces those ideas. That worry or sadness lingers in your mind and can shape future decisions unless you reshape your perception. Your map of reality will always be an interpretation, but it can be an interpretation that helps you rather than hurts you. You can change your map of reality and make it more productive by addressing your thoughts and beliefs and how they impact your behavior.

Thoughts, Core Beliefs, and Behavior

Beliefs are sets of ideas that individuals use to dictate how they'll behave. A belief is something you think is a fact. You feel so strongly about something that you're almost positive it's true, regardless of how well you can prove it. You may have some doubts from time to time, but, overall, you consistently stick to those beliefs. Beliefs are attitudes that you fall back on, because they provide a sense of security, and they make you feel that certain things are constant, which is why something that makes you doubt your beliefs can be so painful. Your beliefs drive your unconscious, habitual behaviors. They become so ingrained in you that they feel natural and inherently true.

When you have trouble managing situations or coping with feelings, you automatically turn to your beliefs for help without exerting too much brainpower. Your beliefs help you determine morality, and they help you decide whether people or things are bad or good. Your whole perspective uses a compilation of your beliefs to fill in the parts of your reality you can't fully understand.

Beliefs are formed based on past experiences and the stimuli around us. Most people's core beliefs— the most driving beliefs they have—are established when they're young children. As they grow older, children commonly challenge the beliefs they've been taught as they begin to think more critically and independently. Nevertheless, many children reaffirm the beliefs they were taught rather than disproving them. As adults, they can challenge these beliefs and, by managing their beliefs, they can create a healthier view of the world that's a more realistic map of reality.

Beliefs can be incredibly powerful. For example, imagine parents telling their children that paperclips are dangerous. Telling a child that paperclips are dangerous seems silly. Nevertheless, when those words go unchallenged, the child will internalize the message, and they might try to avoid paperclips, which could impede their ability to do certain tasks. But as they grow older, the child would likely challenge that belief and overcome the fear of paperclips.

Other beliefs may be harder to debunk. For

instance, if a mom tells her child that dogs are dangerous, the child may become afraid of dogs. This fear could continue into adulthood, because the child has learned to be terrified of dogs. Even rational arguments that dogs aren't something to be scared of may still make it hard for that child to believe. After all, dogs, unlike paperclips, do have the potential to bark and bite. The child would be so convinced by the belief that it would be hard for them to break from that mindset.

You may have beliefs that stand in your way and feel so foundational to who you are that challenging them makes you uncomfortable. Nevertheless, you need to contemplate your limiting beliefs.

While thoughts and beliefs may seem similar, there are some profound differences between them that you must acknowledge if you want to have a complete understanding of how your thoughts and beliefs can make or break your mental health. Thoughts help to form your beliefs. When you have the same thoughts repeatedly, they become beliefs. You become so used to the thoughts that they become ingrained in your subconscious, and it becomes hard to imagine that those thoughts aren't true. Accordingly, when you think negatively, you tend to have a more pessimistic outlook.

Not all thoughts are beliefs. The thoughts that come and go through your mind without repetition never become beliefs. Beliefs are a product of habitual thinking. This means that while it may be hard to break them, you can break them by overwriting those negative thoughts with positive ones, which is a practice that many therapies and techniques discussed in this book use to reduce stress, anxiety, and depression.

As you've seen with the map of reality, perception shapes our views, and it also shapes the way we think. Your thoughts build your beliefs, and your beliefs, in turn, build your sense of what's real. Some of your beliefs will empower you to seek success and find happiness, while others will make the world seem like a dark and scary place with no hope. Try to identify the parts of your belief system that cause you to have negative responses.

Your thought patterns have tremendous power to change your life. The simple act of interrupting negative thought patterns can help you begin to make changes. These changes don't happen overnight, and deeply entrenched beliefs may even take months or years to debunk completely, but, when you focus on the thought patterns you want to instill, you start to question the "truths" you blindly believed.

There will be some beliefs you'll want to keep, and those are ones you can build upon and use to your advantage throughout this process. There's no need to get rid of any belief that's constructive because such beliefs are the ones that help you grow. However, be honest about the beliefs that are hurting you. Many people try to rationalize certain beliefs that they feel psychologically unready to call into question. Open your mind and contemplate, "Is this belief hurting me in covert and manipulative ways?" If you struggle even to pose that question about a particular belief, that belief may be a harmful one.

The way you think isn't something that's out of your control. According to the Massachusetts Institute of Technology (MIT), 45 percent of your daily choices are habitual, meaning they're a product of your subconscious thought patterns and beliefs. You choose what stimuli you feed to your subconscious. When worries or hopelessness begin to fill your head, try saying to yourself, "The world is a place full of opportunity and good things." While it won't feel like saying this is doing anything at first, rewriting your internal monologue can be a powerful first step toward growth.

When you understand how thoughts and core beliefs shape your behaviors, it becomes easier to create a path for growth. You learn that you're in charge of your beliefs, and your thoughts can only have as much control over you as you give them. You may feel helpless against your negative thoughts, but learning to overcome these harmful thoughts and release the power they have over you is the only way to become a happier person. The more you try to avoid the things that make you anxious, stressed, or depressed, the more anxious, stressed, and depressed you'll become.

Cognitive Distortions

While your brain does its best to give you helpful information and create an accurate perception of reality, sometimes it gets a little lost trying to translate what it observes into a sensible perception. Your brain loves to make connections, and sometimes, it will make connections that are overly simplified and don't show the nuance in a situation. This is called a cognitive distortion.

Simple speaking, cognitive distortions are falsehoods that your brain persuades you into believing are true. Cognitive distortions can take a variety of forms, but one common example is polarized thinking. When you think in polarities, you see things as wrong or right, good or bad, or win or lose. After you fail at one task, you may start to think, "I'll fail every task because I can't do anything right." This perception isn't an accurate one, but you become convinced it's true because your brain has pinpointed what it thinks is a pattern.

The problem with cognitive distortions is that they're often shrouded in negativity. They make you expect the worse, and they convince you that you cannot do certain things or that other things are unsafe. Cognitive distortions change your perspective, and they can quickly become harmful to your overall well-being. If you believe false messages, it's hard to make peace with your situation or feel secure. When you feel insecure, your mental health declines, and your doubts start to make it harder to function normally. Anxiety may take hold, and you may feel more stressed as you try to complete tasks. The hardship of your situation may then lead to depression.

Cognitive distortions can also cause you to act in ways that worsen your mental state. For example, someone with an eating disorder may tell themselves, "Not eating helps me," when they lose a couple of pounds. They keep going with harmful behaviors because a faulty pattern was established of believing that an action is "good," even though the behavior, for obvious reasons, is the opposite of helpful.

Likewise, someone with anxiety may say, "Avoiding this task will make me feel calmer," when procrastination only heaps on the pressure and stress of the situation. Delaying the task may have given them a sense of relief before, so they keep doing it. It continues to impair them, but cognitive distortion causes them to keep repeating the same harmful behavior. Cognitive distortions fool you into thinking certain actions are good for you or that they aren't as harmful as they are. Someone may engage in risky behavior and think, "This won't hurt me because it didn't harm me before," when that's not accurate information. People often use these distortions to justify harmful, habitual behaviors that give temporary relief to mental distress, but this causes more problems in the long run.

Negative Thoughts

Negative thoughts can play an influential role in how your brain works because your thoughts help create your map of reality and form your cognitive distortions. It's much easier to give in to negative thoughts than positive ones. People often expect the worst because they're afraid that having hope will lead to disappointment. Negative thoughts are also fueled by the internalization of negative comments that others have made about you in the past. For instance, if your mother tells you that you're ugly, you may start to think you're unattractive until it ultimately becomes a core belief.

Research has shown how much healthier and happier people are when they think positively because the brain responds to the input we give it. So, you can change your outlook by thinking with more positivity. When you think negatively, you're feeding your brain with information it can use against you; therefore, give it information that will help you instead!

The Role of Trauma

Trauma is a significant part of human life, and it can be one of the largest contributors to adverse mental health outcomes, including increased depression, anxiety, and stress. According to the

National Council for Behavioral Health, 70 percent of adults in the United States have experienced at least one traumatic event, which means that 223.4 million people in the United States alone have had trauma. Moreover, among people who seek treatment for mental health issues, 90 percent have gone through trauma. Consequently, if you have trauma, it contributes to some of the issues you may be experiencing.

Trauma is the result of events that cause deep worry or distress. Traumatic experiences are often those that either threaten a person's life or the life or well-being of those they love.

You can have both physical and emotional trauma. Physical trauma can be a response to accidents, injuries, or other physical events. Physical trauma often can trigger emotional trauma, and the scars from emotional trauma often linger longer than those of physical trauma. Trauma can result from physical, verbal, emotional, or sexual abuse, and children who live in violent environments are at an increased risk for trauma. Some people don't realize they have trauma. They might say, "Oh, well, what I went through wasn't that bad compared to other people." However, trauma doesn't mean you were tortured or injured in unthinkable ways. The death of people you love or contracting a serious disease can also cause trauma. Anything can be traumatic if it makes you feel unsafe, so don't downplay those feelings—accept how you feel, even if you don't think it's "that bad."

When you have trauma that you haven't addressed, you're bound to have increased mental challenges. Trauma alone doesn't lead to mental illness, but it's a major contributing factor, and it drives you to rely on unhealthy coping mechanisms that do you more harm than good.

Trauma changes the way you think, which can impact your decision-making processes and your unconscious thoughts. Trauma makes your brain feel unsafe, and when your brain feels unsafe, it focuses on protecting you from future pain, because that pain could threaten your survival. Even in circumstances that don't usually cause anxiety, you may start to feel threatened, even if you can't logically explain why. When you go through trauma, your brain has a stress response, and that stress response reacts to the trauma by changing your future behaviors in an attempt to protect you.

The stress response involves areas of the brain, including the prefrontal cortex, hippocampus, and amygdala. These areas experience lingering changes when they undergo the intense pressure of trauma. As a result, the way your brain processes information shifts when you experience trauma. Your amygdala becomes more active. This part of your brain is responsible for your flight-or-fight reactions and, when it's overactive, it can make you feel as though you're in danger in non-dangerous situations. It stays on guard because it wants to prevent any potential threats from sneaking up on you.

When your amygdala becomes more active, you may be more prone to feeling stressed, and the hippocampus—the part of your brain that handles short-term memories—may become less active. As a result, you may struggle to differentiate between things that happened to you in the past and things that are presently happening.

Finally, the pre-cortex may shrink, and when it does, you have trouble dealing with your emotions and regulating your thoughts. Many of these changes can be found in people who have post-traumatic stress disorder (PTSD), but anyone with trauma can experience them to a lesser degree.

For obvious reasons, trauma makes it hard for you to be mentally healthy, but it also makes it hard for you to be physically healthy. When your physical health declines, this creates additional causes of anxiety, stress, and depression. Thus, not only can your mental health make your physical health worse, but your physical health can make your mental health worse. The Canadian Mental Health Association reports that people with depression are three times as likely to have chronic pain than people without depression. People who have chronic pain are two times as likely to have anxiety or a mood disorder. Mental and physical health are often dependent on one another, which is why the correlations between the two are so important.

According to statistics, you are more likely to experience health issues such as chronic obstructive pulmonary disease (COPD), heart disease, high blood pressure, cancer, and diabetes when you have trauma. These conditions can all reduce your life's quality or longevity, which can then create even more mental unrest. That psychological turbulence can lead to your physical conditions worsening. You can see how these situations can quickly become bleak for those experiencing them. However, by addressing your trauma, you can reduce the potency of some of these issues.

Trauma, unfortunately, is a normal part of life. For many people, it's challenging to manage, but it's nothing to be ashamed of. Using the strategies in this book, you can learn to become conscious of your trauma and take away the power it has to control your life. Simple techniques like listening to music, establishing a healthy diet and exercise routine, practicing meditation, and admitting you have trauma are just some of the most basic techniques you can use to recover.

Recovery from trauma is painful, but it's one of the most important things you can do for your health because working through trauma allows you to heal your brain and teach it new patterns.

Get Professional Help

Before you do anything, you should seek professional help. Seeing a doctor or a mental health professional can help ensure that you have a support system in place to help you improve yourself.

While this book's techniques can help you improve your levels of stress, anxiety, and depression, some people will still need professional support to help push them toward their goals. Additionally, for some people, these issues may be related to their brain chemistry, which may require medication. To have a satisfactory recovery experience, you must take a holistic approach that ensures you achieve long-lasting results and can learn coping skills that will shape the rest of your life.

Recap

Your brain is complex, and it is programmed to keep you safe and make sense of a confusing world. It uses patterns to establish norms, and those norms become the backbone of your behaviors. Your thoughts build into beliefs, and your beliefs create your worldview. Your worldview becomes your map of reality; this map is not always accurate because it's based on your brain's biases and distortions. Your brain loves finding patterns, and sometimes it finds connections that only exist in your head.

When your reality is negative and drives you towards destructive behaviors, you need to question these beliefs and reframe your reality map. It is essential to focus on positive thoughts and vanquish negativity to create better mental health.

Further, you must learn to face the trauma you have endured because trauma changes the activity levels in the important centers of your brain. Your brain is wired to keep you safe, so trying to resist the pattern-seeking nature of your mind is fruitless; instead, you should use the way your brain works to your advantage and feed it with positive stimuli so that you have better mental health.

Finally, I urge you to seek professional help for outstanding issues as part of a holistic approach to curing your mental distress.

CHAPTER 2: MANAGING ANXIETY

What Is Anxiety?

Anxiety affects everyone at some point in their life. However, it can affect some people more than others, to the point where it becomes disabling. Most people don't recognize their anxiety for what it is and instead think there's something "wrong" with them. Some people are preoccupied with the symptoms of anxiety (e.g., stomachaches, increased heart rate, shortness of breath, etc.) without realizing the cause. Others think they're weird, weak, or even going crazy. Unfortunately, these thoughts only make people feel even more anxious and self-conscious.

As awful as it can be, anxiety is a normal part of life that can arise at any time. Even if you don't have an anxiety disorder, you've probably experienced anxiety at some point. Whether you have an anxiety disorder or anxiety that only pops up now and then, anxiety can be painful and debilitating whenever it shows up. To effectively manage anxiety, you need to better understand what it is and how to combat it.

Types of Anxiety Disorders

Anxiety disorders are the most common mental health issue. Around the world, an estimated 284 million people have anxiety disorders. There are six commonly specified anxiety disorders, but you can have life-altering anxiety without being diagnosed with one of these conditions, which are discussed below. Everyone deserves relief from their anxiety, no matter how severe it is.

44

General Anxiety Disorder

General anxiety disorder (GAD) is defined as an overabundance of worry or anxiety experienced by an individual for at least half a year for most days of the week. This sense of fear can relate to any number of things, including career, family life, health, or routines. People who have general anxiety disorder often feel worried about a wide range of things, and these fears are destructive to their well-being.

The common symptoms and signs of this disorder include restlessness and a feeling that you have excess nervous energy. You may also feel exhausted more easily because even doing basic tasks can cause a highly anxious response. If you have this type of anxiety, you may have difficulty thinking clearly. When the anxiety takes hold, you may have trouble accessing memories in your panicked state because of how the brain reacts to fear. You may become moodier because you feel on edge all the time, and your feelings of anxiety

45

may seem like they're uncontrollable and volatile. Your anxiety can have other impacts, too, such as making it hard for you to get to sleep, stay asleep, or have good-quality sleep, and it can make your body feel achy and tense.

When you have GAD, you may feel powerless against your worry. Going through your daily routine may feel stressful and dangerous, no matter how hard you try to resist your anxious feelings. The truth is, you can't ignore your anxiety. To make it go away, you have to face your worries and acknowledge them because, if you don't, they'll always be the monster that could be hiding in your closet. Challenging your fears may show you the monster was never there to begin with or that the monster isn't as dangerous as you thought!

Panic Disorder

Panic disorder is a condition in which people have repeating episodes of panic attacks that they do not expect. Panic attacks are instances when you have extreme fear that often comes with startling symptoms. These attacks happen suddenly, and they often reach their worst severity in a few minutes. Nevertheless, they are hard to manage, and they can cause increased mental illness.

Some of the symptoms of a panic attack can be truly scary. As your heart starts to pound loud and fast in your chest and ears, you may start to feel sweat running down your back or your hands becoming clammy. You may begin to shake uncontrollably or tremble. During a panic attack, you may have trouble catching your breath or feel like you can't take sufficiently deep breaths. You may also feel everything around you is going wrong and can't be fixed, even though you don't know why you feel that way. Your feelings and worries will become overwhelming, and you may struggle to tame them.

Panic disorder can be terrifying because you may

feel like you're dying when you experience panic episodes. People who experience panic attacks for the first time or who don't realize what panic attacks are may think a panic attack is a heart attack or another serious physical condition. The fear that they may be dying only intensifies the episode and makes it harder for them to calm down. When you have a panic attack, you may worry you'll have these terrifying episodes indefinitely, and that fear can interfere with your plans and reduce your quality of life.

Agoraphobia

Agoraphobia is the fear of one or more of the following specific activities: the use of public transportation, being outside of your home by yourself, waiting in a line or standing in a crowd, or having to be in enclosed or open spaces. Agoraphobia can be a debilitating condition because it makes you avoid normal activities you may want to do but feel afraid to try.

When you have agoraphobia, you may feel unable to leave your house. Although you want to go out and do things with your loved ones, there's a mental barrier that stands in your way. Further, you may be embarrassed about the responses your agoraphobia causes, such as extreme panic and other symptoms for which other people, who are unaware of how anxiety manifests, might judge you. While agoraphobia isn't something you should feel ashamed of, many people do. The best way to get your life back on track is to address your fears.

Specific Phobias

A phobia is a fear of a specific thing or multiple things. Some common phobias include heights, flying, animals or bugs, and needles. It's normal to be afraid of a growling dog that you don't know or a Black Widow spider in your closet, but when you have a phobia, the fear you feel is taken to the point of irrationality. That doesn't mean you're an irrational person; it only means your brain is overresponding to a potential threat.

Phobias can result from past experiences or distorted perceptions of situations. Even a parent expressing something like, "That dog is mean and attacks people," can make a child start to be afraid of all dogs (a cognitive distortion). While it might be rational for that child to be tentative around unknown dogs, when a person is phobic of dogs, they become phobic of *all* dogs. More than that, they may not even be able to walk by a fence that has a dog behind it. Whereas nonphobic people would feel safe, someone with a fear of dogs might persistently worry that the dog will jump over the fence and attack them. Thus, phobias can cause people to avoid situations and worry incessantly about unlikely circumstances. Someone afraid of spiders might be frightened to look inside their closet because of how intense their fear is, which shows how extreme a specific phobia can become.

People who have phobias may have trouble

accomplishing everyday activities. They may feel shame about their fears because while they can't help their reactions, they often know their responses aren't typical.

Phobias aren't something you need to be ashamed of and, with treatment, you can lessen them or even cure them. It's best to address your phobias because usually, they only get worse over time if not dealt with.

Social Anxiety Disorder

Social anxiety is defined as a reoccurring sense of fear in social situations. Social anxiety doesn't mean you're introverted or hate people (although that can be the case). People with social anxiety don't avoid social situations because they don't want to be social. Their avoidance stems from a fear of what will happen when they try to speak or interact with other people. You may want to do certain things, but your anxiety prevents you from doing them. As a result, social anxiety can rob you of so much and make you feel you can't function like a normal human being.

People with social anxiety may struggle to go out in public and form relationships with other people. They may become uncomfortable in large groups or worry they're being judged when interacting with other people. People with this disorder may avoid going to social functions because of how intense their fears are. They also commonly ruminate about social situations, replaying certain encounters in their heads. When you have social anxiety, you may feel isolated because you choose to spend time alone rather than challenging your fears. You may worry that people would never like you if they got to know you, so you keep to yourself while yearning for human connection. Social anxiety may do more than just impede your social life. It can also make it hard to advance your career or work in certain jobs. Thus, while social anxiety may seem like shyness or aloofness to the untrained eye, it's a serious condition that hurts millions of people.

Separation Anxiety Disorder

Generally, separation anxiety disorder is something that young children experience, but adults can experience this in some circumstances. When you have this disorder, you're afraid of being detached or separated from important people in your life. You may persistently fear that something will take a particular person away from you, commonly a caregiver or someone you emotionally rely on. People with this condition spend much time worrying that the person they're attached to will die, leave them, or otherwise be separated from them. They may have nightmares or physical symptoms of upset when distant from the person at the center of their anxiety.

Causes of Anxiety

There's no one cause of anxiety because every case is different. However, many people experience overlap in their anxiety symptoms and causes.

53

Below are some of the common sources of anxiety.

- Stress - stressors such as an increased load at work, chaos at home, or other environmental factors can often trigger anxiety.

- Trauma - whether emotional, sexual, or physical.

- Substance abuse - Drug or alcohol use or misuse or withdrawal can cause or worsen anxiety. Even something as simple as coffee can make you feel jittery or nervous when you drink too much of it. Or, if you have coffee every day, not having it can make you feel equally anxious.

- Personality - people with certain personality types are more prone to anxiety disorders than others.

- Your DNA - people who have family members with anxiety are at a higher risk of having it themselves.

- Other medical conditions and symptoms may also make you feel anxious. For example, if you have irritable bowel syndrome, frequent or painful bowel movements may make you feel anxious in public because of the potential embarrassment that comes with IBS. Intense medical procedures or terminal illnesses can also commonly contribute to anxiety.

There's no limit to the number of causes of your anxiety, but, in most cases, anxiety is caused by a combination of several factors.

How Anxiety Affects You

While many people know about the impact of anxiety on mental health, fewer people are aware of the physical symptoms, including issues with the digestive, cardiovascular, urinary, and respiratory systems. Anxiety can significantly affect the body, and longstanding anxiety

55

increases the risk of developing chronic physical conditions. You may start to feel headaches, nausea, digestive issues, body aches, and other symptoms caused by your fear response. Further, people with anxiety are more prone to health conditions such as high blood pressure, heart disease, or diabetes.

Everyone has anxiety from time to time, but an anxiety disorder can degrade your quality of life. This is largely due to the psychological and physiological impacts it has on you over time. Every day you continue to have anxiety, you're limiting how much you can do and, most importantly, you're limiting how good you can feel about your life, yourself, and even those around you. Your worry may feel like it's keeping you safe, but you put the things you cherish the most in danger when you spend so much time worrying.

Your anxiety may make you feel bad about yourself. You may start to doubt your worth and role in your own life. Anxiety can also cause strain on your relationships and make it hard for you to communicate with people you love. Feelings of moodiness and insecurity can often cause relationship issues when they aren't handled. When you have anxiety in one area of your life, it starts to spread to other areas. Consequently, anxiety can have far-reaching impacts on your life that you can't afford to ignore.

Overcoming Anxiety

There are many ways to overcome your anxiety, but it's crucial to remember that everyone is different, and you should choose what works best for you. The first thing you should do is seek treatment. Therapists are great choices if you're looking for a professional who can help you work through contributing issues and give you the coping skills you need to get better. Further, don't be afraid of pharmaceutical treatment. Some people have chemical imbalances that make it hard for them to address their anxiety without medication. Medication is sometimes an essential part of treatment, and taking it doesn't make you weak-willed. If someone took medication for a physical ailment, you wouldn't think they were weak, so you shouldn't believe that about yourself and your condition either!

Question what your anxiety tells you. Don't just give in to the anxious thoughts and assume they're true because, for the most part, your internal conversations at that moment are exaggerations of the truth. When you start to question what your anxiety is saying, you start to break the cognitive distortions you've created.

Use visualization to imagine yourself as a calmer person. Imagining yourself in the mental state you'd like to have is an invaluable technique that allows you to create better results. Just close your eyes and imagine that the weight of your anxiety is falling off you and is dissipating into the air around you.

Remember that change takes time, and setbacks aren't failures. When you have bad days, it doesn't mean you're not making progress. You're still making progress even when certain days don't go as well as you'd like them to go. Thus, when you have bad days or moments, take them in stride and learn to use them to help you improve in the future. When anxiety spikes in your life after being quiet for a while, it has nothing to do with how hard you've worked to address it, and it doesn't define your success. Anxiety happens, and while you can limit when and how much it happens, being sometimes unable to stop it is normal and doesn't mean you've failed.

Getting Over Social Anxiety

Social anxiety can interfere with every part of your life, but there are ways you can overcome it and improve your ability to interact in social situations. Don't miss out on time with friends or loved ones; instead, make more time for what you love and less time for worrying. Don't try to find ways to avoid your fears. Instead, learn how to confront them. As you face your fears and survive social situations, you'll start to realize that the things you were afraid of weren't as dangerous as you made them out to be.

Don't avoid social interactions. As counterintuitive as it sounds, you can't keep avoiding social interactions because when you try to avoid social situations, you deprive yourself of happiness and validate your fears. When you avoid something, you don't make it go away; you only further convince yourself that whatever you're afraid of is worth being afraid of. When you commit to social events, you challenge yourself, and you learn to use coping skills, which are crucial if you want to get better. Practice makes perfect, so you must practice being social to diminish your social anxiety.

Recognize when you need to take a moment to yourself, and be honest with other people about your needs. While it's good to push yourself, you'll need to take mental breaks every so often to reorient and ward off any bubbling panic. Learn to figure out how you feel when you're becoming overwhelmed and when you're with others, be honest with them and tell them when you need a moment alone or when you need to go home. Push yourself as hard as you can, but don't push yourself so hard that you do more harm than good.

Celebrate your progress because you deserve to take pride in what you've accomplished. When you make progress, you need to appreciate it. Doing so will reinforce the idea that what you're doing is good and rewarding. Train your brain to believe that resisting anxiety is something that should feel good. When you do that, you'll defy your social anxiety more easily because your brain will learn to associate your progress with reward. You can celebrate with friends or celebrate with self-care tactics or hobbies, but mark your progress with some rewarding behavior.

For more information on becoming more sociable and confident in social settings, I recommend my book: *"How to be Charismatic, Develop Confidence, and Exude Leadership: The Miracle Formula for Magnetic Charisma, Defeating Anxiety, and Winning at Communication."*

Managing Panic Attacks

Panic attacks come without much warning, but you can still learn to manage them and reduce their frequency. Some people can even eliminate panic attacks entirely or almost completely.

The first thing you need to do is know the signs of a panic attack and, more specifically, learn how your body responds when you're having such an episode. It can help to write down your experiences when you have a panic attack, so you can start to seek patterns and be more aware of what's happening to you.

Don't limit your behavior to trying to avoid panic attacks; acknowledge your feelings of panic rather than trying to ignore them. Focus on how you're feeling at that moment. Live your life in the ways that help you feel happier and healthier even if you worry that a panic attack may result. Instead of worrying about how or when a panic attack might strike if you do a particular thing, focus on the enjoyment you have doing that thing. Trying to control when panic attacks strike isn't helpful because the more you try to ignore your problem and push it away, the harder it becomes to change.

If you feel a panic attack coming on, take deep breaths and, if you can't seem to focus, use grounding techniques. You can ground yourself by counting as you breathe. You can also focus on your surroundings and your various sensory processes. For example, suppose you're in someone else's house and feeling anxious. In that case, you can try to identify all the red items (or any color or quality) in the room. If you're in a busy food court, you can try to identify all the smells around you. Try to be specific with the focus of your grounding techniques, so look for something red rather than something that's just reddish-orange. Focus on what's going on now rather than letting your panic pull you into the past or future.

Be aware of feelings such as hunger, anger, loneliness, and tiredness (H.A.L.T.). These can all be triggers for your panic attacks. When you start to feel panic-attack symptoms, consider whether you may be experiencing one of those four things, and then try to address it.

Further, it would be best if you were careful using substances that alter your brain's functioning, such as drugs, alcohol, caffeine, and nicotine. These substances can also trigger panic. Learn what tends to trigger you the most. Increased awareness can help you get your panic under control.

10 Exercises for Managing Anxiety

Below are a few easy techniques you can start right now to start managing your anxiety.

1. Take calming breaths. When you start to feel overwhelmed, begin taking deep breaths. As you focus on your breathing, your anxiety will begin to lessen.

2. Listening to music is another excellent calming technique that can help you relax and alleviate anxious thoughts.

3. Close your eyes for a few moments. This task seems so simple, but because 80 percent of the stimuli you take in is processed via your vision, closing your eyes can help you get in touch with your other senses while avoiding overstimulation.

4. Acknowledge what's bothering you. Learning to find language to express your anxiety helps you process it.

5. Go for a walk in Nature. Walks help improve your cardiovascular health, but they also improve your mental state too. When you go for a walk, especially in Nature, it gives you a chance to think and escape the business of your life.

6. Talk to someone about your struggles. When you don't know what else to do, it can feel good to talk to someone about what's bothering you. It relieves some of your burdens and, when you share your anxiety, it becomes less shameful.

7. Find a hobby that allows you to express some of the emotions you've been withholding.

8. Take time to yourself if you need it. If you feel you need a moment alone, find a way to relax, and give yourself a little TLC.

9. Practice journaling and write down your feelings. When you write down what you're feeling, you learn to express your anxiety in new ways, giving it less power over you.

10. Remember that you're not your anxiety. You're so much more than your fears. Remember all the things that make you who you are despite your anxiety.

Recap

Anxiety is your fear response taken to an extreme. It makes you worry persistently about things that are not healthy to worry about. It's important to distinguish that anxiety is not a normal fear, but it can be a response to cognitive distortions being created during fearful events.

There are several types of anxiety disorders, such as general anxiety, social anxiety, agoraphobia, specific phobias, panic disorder, and separation anxiety. However, you may also experience anxiety that doesn't reach the level of a disorder, and that anxiety is still important to address.

Anxiety can be caused by many factors, including genetic, cultural, and environmental factors, which means that it can impact anyone. It is usually not the result of a single cause. It often relies on cognitive distortions and other false perceptions.

Anxiety inevitably impacts the level of functioning you have in social, romantic, professional, and personal situations, and it can cause both psychological and physical symptoms. While it feels bleak and uncontrollable, you can use strategies to overcome and manage your anxiety. With simple exercises, you can start to feel better in a matter of days.

CHAPTER 3: REDUCING STRESS

What Is Stress?

According to the American Institute of Stress, 77 percent of people have experienced a stress level that repeatedly caused them to have physical symptoms of stress. In comparison, 73 percent of those people consistently had psychological impacts. Those numbers are around three-quarters of the United States population, which shows how common stress is. A startling one-third of the population reported that their stress was extreme.

Stress is a global problem, but it impacts certain populations more than others. Unfortunately, stress not only hurts individuals, it hurts society at large. Statistics show that stress is a widespread problem that only threatens to worsen if we don't change our relationship with our work and aspects of our personal lives.

You've probably experienced feelings of stress, but you may not fully understand what it is. Stress is your body's natural response to situations you perceive as dangerous. When you feel stress, chemicals are released by your brain that cause physical reactions such as increased heartbeat and intensified breathing. Epinephrine rushes through your body and causes a fight-or-flight response. When those chemical surges recur frequently, they can result in side effects such as insomnia, anxiety, headaches, or stroke.

Stress shares similar processes with anxiety, but stress is more about what you're currently dealing with rather than being caused by thinking about the future. Many people who have stress also have anxiety, which can feel similar but isn't precisely the same. The American Psychological Association explains that you don't need a stressor when you have anxiety, but stress usually has an event or thing that externally triggers it. Therefore, stress is based on short-term causes, but it can become chronic as triggers add up.

Anything that causes worry or pressure in your life can cause stress. One of the most common causes is the work we do. The American Institute of Stress says a mere six percent of all workers don't feel stressed when they're at work, while 83 percent of workers feel stressed *because* of work. Each day, one million workers don't go to work because of the stress they experience in their workplace.

Another major cause of stress is financial problems. The American Psychological

Association says 77 percent of people experience financial worries. People are also highly stressed about their families and the health of themselves and their loved ones. While these statistics are U.S.-centric, most of these concerns are echoed in counties like Greece (the country with the highest reported daily stress levels), Canada, Australia, France, the United Kingdom, and most other countries worldwide.

Stress impacts you in many ways. Just under 50 percent of people say their stress keeps them awake at night. Stress doesn't just make you feel bad; it makes it hard to focus on the tasks you need to do. Stress can lead to depression, anxiety, and physical ailments like heart disease, diabetes, and high blood pressure. Estimates suggest that workplace stress causes over 100,000 deaths per year, and the related healthcare costs are $190 billion per year. The cost of stress isn't something we can afford to take lightly.

Stress also commonly causes a chain reaction in which each symptom makes the other symptoms worse. For example, your job may lead to you having stress. As you have more stress, your blood pressure goes up. As your blood pressure goes up, you become stressed about your health in addition to the stress you have about your work. It becomes harder to work with all that stress, and you find yourself becoming more anxious about everything you have to do. The stress makes your brain fuzzier, so your work quality diminishes, and your boss gets on your case about improving. You begin to fight with your partner over small things because you bring the worry from work home, and the strain hurts your relationship, which—you guessed it—adds more stress. To deal with all the stress, you may turn to a coping tool like eating junk food. While junk food is okay in moderation, you may start to use it as a crutch and not meet your proper dietary requirements. The nutritional deficiency can then worsen your blood pressure and increase your odds of developing other conditions like diabetes or heart disease. Those conditions may put you in the hospital, tearing you away from your family and work. As you can see, stress can quickly spiral out of control.

Types of Stress

Knowing what type of stress you have can help you understand its nature and the kind of role it plays in your life. You may have experienced all of the following at some point, but focus on the type of stress you have right now.

Acute Stress

We all experience acute stress at some time in our life. When you're in an unfamiliar situation that you aren't entirely sure how to manage, you'll feel stress. This sort of stress isn't always a bad thing. For example, this type of stress can be that exhilarated but slightly on-edge feeling you have when you're on a roller coaster. Most moments of acute stress aren't that harmful, but they can cause severe acute stress, which can occur in

74

PTSD and other mental-health conditions. Acute stress can be okay if it's healthy and helps you grow and experience exciting new things.

Episodic Acute Stress

If you have episodic acute stress, this means you have acute stress often. This stress is often caused by anxiety and worrying about what might come around the corner. It can also make you feel like you're always dealing with obstacles and give you the impression you're living far too chaotically. Certain people are more prone to this kind of stress. For example, emergency service workers and other people who have high-intensity jobs may have more episodic acute stress, because they're in so many situations that may trigger a stress response. With this stress type, episodes of stress come and go, but they pop up more frequently than with acute stress.

Chronic Stress

Chronic stress means your stress levels are high

for a long time. This type of stress is harmful to your health, and it can cause both lasting physical and psychological symptoms. Chronic stress wears you down, and it may make you feel you're never secure.

Managing Stress

Stress is a natural part of life and, while you can't always control every situation, you can control how you respond to it. When stress becomes overwhelming, it can take a toll on your overall health. That's why it's vital to have effective stress-management techniques that can calm your mind and body.

The more you practice stress-management techniques, the more they'll become second nature to you. You'll learn to deal with stress as it happens, and you won't have to think too hard about how to respond.

The following are some suggestions to help you manage stress:

Take charge of the situations that stress you out. When you experience a stressful situation, face it head-on because you make the situation more stressful if you try to ignore or avoid it. Communicate your stress to other people. If your spouse or friend is doing something that stresses you out, that's something you can have a conversation about. It's okay to admit your stress. You might not get the outcome you want by talking it out, but people are usually willing to meet you halfway to find a solution that works for both of you. If you don't communicate your stress, you put yourself at a handicap because you aren't using all the available tools.

Don't let yourself get bored. You need to keep your mind stimulated and give yourself something worthwhile to do when you start to feel restless. When you allow yourself to become bored, it may seem like something is wrong, especially if you're used to being busy.

Create incremental goals. Most people fail to create incremental goals, which causes them to feel overwhelmed. Incremental goals are small goals that build up to a larger one. Instead of saying your goal is to lose 40 pounds, you can say you want to lose two pounds per week for 20 weeks. When you complete a task incrementally, it feels less abstract, and it becomes less stressful. If you have a project that causes you to stress, break it into smaller pieces, and tackle one part at a time. By doing that, you can celebrate small accomplishments and keep your mind at ease.

Dealing with Stress at Work

You need to pay special attention to workplace stress because it's one of the most prevalent forms, and it's a kind of stress that you bring home with you. Inevitably, work will cause some degree of stress, but that stress doesn't have to become chronic if you have the right coping strategies.

Schedule dedicated leisure time. If you have a whole pile of work on your desk that you need to get done on a tight deadline, taking time for leisure can seem impossible, but the truth is, when you don't take time for leisure, you won't be as productive while you work. By taking just a tiny bit of time to do something you enjoy, you can decompress. Then, when you return to your work, you can work more efficiently. What you do in your leisure time is up to you, but leisure is essential to your well-being. People who take the time to relax live longer and are happier.

Practice problem-solving. If you can hone your problem-solving skills, you can go into challenging situations feeling less pressure. The idea is to approach issues with a problem-solving mindset. Next time a problem arises at work, ask yourself. "How can I solve this?" rather than thinking of all the things that could go wrong.

Challenge negative thoughts. When the negative thoughts you have about yourself or your work start to get you down, confront those thoughts. When you have a negative thought, it doesn't get you anywhere good, so try to add positive thoughts to your internal dialogue. Say, "I made this mistake, but I have many skills I can use to solve this problem." When you learn to challenge those negative thoughts, it's easier to find mental peace.

For more information on effectively managing negative thoughts and emotions, I recommend my book: "How to Stop Being Negative, Angry, and Mean: Master Your Mind and Take Control of Your Life."

Learn to manage your time more efficiently, so you can get more done in less time. Time management is one of the most important things you can do to address your stress because when you learn to manage your time, you feel confident you have the time you need to accomplish your tasks. Time management gives you one less thing that could cause stress. Keep in mind that good time management includes leaving time for unexpected issues because problems always come up, no matter how well you plan.

Acupressure for Stress

Acupressure involves applying pressure to various "pressure points" on your body to soothe your tension. With your thumb or index finger, you can place gentle pressure on these spots:

- The "hall of impression" point – This point is located in the middle of your forehead between your eyes.
- The "union valley" point - This point is located between your thumb and index finger.
- The "great surge" point – This point is located between your big toe and second toe.

- The "heavenly gate" point – This point is located in the middle of the upper portion of your outer ear.

- The "inner frontier gate" point – This point is located in the middle of the back of your forearm, about an inch and a half above your wrist.

- The "shoulder well" point – This point is located in your shoulder muscle. If you're pregnant, you shouldn't use this point because it can induce labor.

These locations are all known for their stress-reducing properties, and acupressure is an easy way to decrease the tension in your body.

11 Amazing Stress Relief Techniques

1. Meditation is a known stress reliever because it helps you stay present and reminds you to focus on your inner processes and what you need to accomplish. You can find thousands of free

or paid meditation programs, or you can practice self-guided meditation.

2. Breathing; just as it does for anxiety, breathing also helps with stress.

3. Practice Gratitude. Determine what you are grateful for each day. People who show gratitude tend to be healthier, and they have lower stress levels. When you can find things you are thankful to have, you stop focusing on the bad and start appreciating the good.

4. Set boundaries and be realistic about what you can achieve, not just physically but emotionally as well. Boundaries are a way for you to express the things that make you comfortable or uncomfortable, or what you would like to happen or not happen within your relationships. If you don't think that

you can complete an assignment on time, be honest with your boss about your needs.

5. Laugh more. The old proverb that says that laughter is the best medicine is pretty spot on. A study showed that people who laughed more tended to be less stressed. This response to laughter is because laughter has the opposite impacts on your body as stress, and it naturally relaxes your mind and tense muscles. When you are feeling down or stressed, watch your favorite comedies, watch comedy specials, anything that is going to get you laughing in a genuine, carefree manner.

6. Chewing gum is a simple way to relieve stress. One study suggested that when people chewed gum, they were less stressed. Another study indicated that people had more relief when they chewed more firmly! So, chew away! But be

warned, chomping too loud may stress out the people around you.

7. Ask a loved one for a hug. When someone hugs you, your body releases the chemical oxytocin, which is linked to being happier and less stressed. Simple acts of physical affection can do wonders for your stress levels.

8. Various studies have connected stress management and aromatherapy. Aromatherapy or essential oil therapy is a holistic healing treatment that uses natural plant extracts to balance your mood and arouse overall well-being. Some of the common plants used in this process are rosemary, sandalwood, ylang-ylang, thyme, and lavender.

9. Get in touch with your artistic side. Drawing or painting can be a cathartic

process that helps you express your feelings in a non-pressuring manner. Even if you don't consider yourself to be good at artistic pursuits, drawing or other artistic activities may make you feel better.

10. Watch out for sugary foods and caffeine. Research shows that you may start to feel more stressed and anxious if you have too much caffeine. Further, if you eat sugar, you have high energy levels that crash and leave you feeling tired. That exhaustion puts you at a higher risk for stress. Further, most sugary foods aren't nutritionally dense, so they do not provide your body with the materials it needs for peak functionality. Both caffeine and sugar can also interfere with your sleep, again making you more prone to stress.

11. Prioritize the parts of your life that make you feel calm. If work stresses you out,

spend less time focusing on work. Instead, focus on whatever it is that makes you happy because those are the things that will help you go to work with a clear mind.

Recap

Stress is a normal bodily response that helps you manage life-threatening or seemingly dangerous situations. Billions of people experience stress each day, and for those with chronic stress, stress can be incredibly debilitating. Even so, episodic acute stress or acute stress can still be harmful, and it can help to learn coping skills to manage all kinds of stress. Stress causes physical and mental issues that have lasting impacts on your well-being. While there is no one cause for stress, work-related stress is one of the most prevalent globally, followed by stress related to finances, family life, health, etc. Nearly anything can cause stress, but with a few simple strategies, such as acupressure, deep breathing, leisure activities, and time management, you can begin to rectify the problems that stress causes.

CHAPTER 4: DEFYING DEPRESSION

What is Depression?

Depression is a mood disorder characterized by persistent feelings of sadness that make everyday interactions and tasks difficult, if not impossible. When you have depression, you have a lowered mood. While many people experience it as deep, prolonged sadness, that's not always the case because depression manifests in a myriad of ways. When you have depression, you don't feel like yourself; you may feel sad, but you may also feel empty, restless, or numb. You may feel detached from yourself and feel like you're taking a back seat in your own life rather than being the driver.

Depression can cause you to isolate and avoid social interactions, and it can make you feel you don't have the energy or desire to accomplish things you used to want to do. In many ways, depression feels like living in a gray haze to those who suffer it, and this gray haze can make you feel hopeless if you don't treat it.

Depression, as it worsens, not only causes your quality of life to decrease, but it can also result in harmful thoughts that can become destructive. If you continue to feel down or hopeless, you may start to engage in self-harm. You may have suicidal ideations, which can lead to suicide attempts and, possibly, suicide. Tragically, when one person commits suicide, it can cause a "suicide contagion," meaning people exposed to suicidal behavior become more at risk. Depression and its terrible consequences can spread, which only points out that this a severe condition that must be dealt with seriously.

Diagnosis and Symptoms

There's a stark medical difference between feelings of sadness and clinical depression. While some people may feel depressed, professionals use specific diagnostic criteria to diagnose various types of depression. These criteria can include symptoms, intensity, and duration of depression. These factors are essential to your treatment. It's recommended that a professional diagnose depression, because there are a number of complex conditions that fall under the depression umbrella. For those seeking to understand depression better, it's more useful to look at the full collection of symptoms that most often occur during depression. Still, you should always keep in mind that each individual experiences these symptoms differently or may only experience a few.

The most prominent aspect of depression is a declined mood, but evaluating your other symptoms can help you differentiate a normal period of feeling blue from clinical depression. A major sign that you may have depression is if you stop finding joy in things that formerly evoked passion. You may start to feel numb or restless. You may also feel guilt, hopelessness, and sadness. It may become harder for you to pay attention to tasks, and you may ruminate, focusing on the same thought repetitively.

Intense fatigue, regardless of how well you sleep, is another symptom. Some people may have insomnia, while others will sleep longer than usual. Your appetite may change, becoming excessive or deficient, which can cause weight changes. You may start to cry a lot, or you may feel more anxious. These symptoms are some of the most prevalent, but depression can manifest in other ways as well.

Also, different groups of people experience depression in unique ways that shift the way symptoms present themselves. Men and women may experience depression differently based on social standards. For example, a man's moodiness when he's depressed may cause him to be angrier or more aggressive, while moodiness caused by depression in a woman may make her more irritable. Children also experience symptoms in slightly different ways. They may be more prone to excessive crying and feeling they can't do anything right; they may also have more behavioral issues in school or with siblings.

Additionally, depression can worsen the symptoms of preexisting conditions. If you have heart disease, diabetes, asthma, arthritis, or cancer, your depression can make it harder to fight these conditions and can cause responses in your body that make the symptoms more unbearable. These are just some of the conditions that depression can directly impact. Indirectly, depression can deteriorate any condition you have, because it makes it tougher to do basic things (sleeping, eating healthy, exercise, etc.) that are needed to improve your health.

Types of Depression

There are several types of depression that can impact people in a wide range of ways, and they can have a wide range of triggers.

Major Depression

Major depressive disorder (MDD) is the type of depression that comes to mind when most people think of depression. When you have this type of depression, you feel depressed most or all days of the week for a large chunk of your day. You'll probably have symptoms that are more outwardly recognizable. You may have no interest in tending to personal hygiene, so you may not brush your teeth or comb your hair, and you may have difficulty getting out of bed and starting your day. You may be diagnosed with this condition if you have at least five of the following symptoms that occur for at least two weeks:

- A depressed mood or loss of interest in pleasurable activities
- Suicidal thoughts
- Fatigue
- Struggling to focus or make decisions
- Low sense of worth or high levels of guilt
- Lacking in vigor or vitality
- Lacking in spirit or interest
- Sleep issues
- Weight gain or loss

Persistent Depressive Disorder

When you experience depression for two years or more, you have what's known as persistent depressive disorder (PDD). This disorder combines symptoms from the diagnoses of chronic major depressive disorder and dysthymia. When you have this disorder, you generally experience the same usual symptoms of depression, but these symptoms are less severe and persist for more extended periods. While the symptoms may be less intense, that doesn't mean they're less important or that you can ignore them. These symptoms can make you appear "functional" when, in actuality, you struggle to do typical and enjoyable things. Because it's chronic, this type of depression can make it harder for you to handle your symptoms. You usually experience this condition starting as a child or teenager, and it can have some overlap with other forms of depression. For example, those with PDD may still experience spells of major depression.

Bipolar Disorder, AKA "Manic Depression"

Bipolar disorder is a mood disorder that causes people to experience swings between mania and depression. They go from feeling high to feeling low, and these sudden changes are intense. Because manic depression is a distinct disorder, the medical and therapeutic approaches to treating this condition are different from treating other types of depression. For example, antidepressants haven't proven to be effective for bipolar disorder and, among a small percentage of people, they may even worsen manic symptoms. These fundamental differences show how important it is to not only be able to identify that you have depression but to know the cause of it.

Seasonal Affective Disorder

People who have seasonal affective disorder (SAD) tend to have depression during the winter months, because there's less sunlight during winter. SAD will start to lessen as the sun begins to come out more and the days become longer. When you have this disorder, traditional treatment options for depression can help, but you may also want to consider adding supplemental light therapy, which uses a special lamp to simulate sunlight.

Psychotic Depression

Psychotic depression is a severe type of depression. People who have this type exhibit typical major depressive symptoms, but they also have psychotic symptoms. The psychotic symptoms can include delusions or hallucinations. These psychotic symptoms usually align with the negative thought patterns of the individual's depression (for example, the feeling of "I can't do anything right" can lead to thinking that people are mocking you). Again, if you have this type of depression, the diagnosis will determine the exact nature of treatment you need.

Postpartum Depression

Postpartum (peripartum) depression is a subtype of major depression. It's experienced after a woman has given birth and is treated in much the same way as major depression. Knowing the cause can provide clinicians with a better idea of what's happening psychologically.

Premenstrual Dysphoric Disorder (PMDD)

Some women experience depressive symptoms whenever they start their periods. They commonly experience a depressed mood, mood swings, increased anxiety levels, and changes in sleep and appetite. This type of depression can be treated using therapeutic approaches and antidepressants or birth-control pills, which regulate the hormones that cause the symptoms.

Situational Depression

While this isn't an official diagnosis, many people may experience depressed moods that are significant but are influenced mostly by situational factors. This form of depression is triggered by high-stress situations. You can benefit from techniques learned in treatments like cognitive behavioral therapy (CBT), which we will discuss in the next chapter.

Atypical Depression

Like situational depression, atypical depression isn't an official diagnosis. One of the main characteristics of atypical depression that distinguishes it from major depression is mood responsiveness. The person with atypical depression will see their mood improve if something positive happens. In major depression, positive changes will rarely bring on an improvement in mood.

<u>Causes of Depression</u>

Depression can be caused by various factors, and often it is caused by multiple things happening at once. People who have a family history of mood disorders are more at risk of depression. Additionally, people who have less active frontal lobes are more prone to depression. Both of these tendencies suggest both genetic and neurological risk factors are essential in the development of depression. Further, those who've abused substances also have a greater risk of depression;

100

among those who abuse substances, 21 percent are depressed.

If you have medical conditions such as chronic pain or other disorders that add complications to your life, you're also more likely to become depressed. The same is true of mental-health conditions. Mental illnesses such as eating disorders, obsessive-compulsive disorder, and anxiety often occur with depression. Depression can also be caused by traumatic experiences like childhood trauma, abuse, or the death of a loved one.

The causes of depression aren't simple to trace, and they usually have complex roots. Those complex roots can be just one of the challenges you face when trying to address your depression.

Treating Depression

While symptoms of depression may ease on their own, depression can lead to harmful behaviors and a lower quality of life. Treatment is the best choice. It can help reduce symptoms more quickly, and it can give you the skills to resist future depression.

Depression treatment often uses multiple methods at once to address contributing issues and chemical imbalances in the brain. The treatment is customized to the patient's needs, so it requires psychological and medical consultations. The use of medications such as antidepressants, selective serotonin reuptake inhibitors (SSRIs), and antipsychotics along with modalities such as psychotherapy and CBT is common. Not everyone will need medication, and the exact formula will depend on the type of depression, causes, and other medical factors that may influence the treatment.

Alternative Therapies

While you should always seek a professional when you suspect you have depression, experts often encourage using integrative therapies in addition to Western medicine. When treating depression, there are several treatments you can use to improve some of your symptoms.

Reflexology is a practice that involves a practitioner applying pressure to different points on the foot that correspond to particular areas on the body. Some people turn to acupuncture for help. This technique developed in ancient China involves the placement of needles by an acupuncturist at specific points on your body. Herbal remedies like Ginkgo Biloba and St. John's wort are commonly used. Massage therapy, mediation, and yoga are other popular techniques used to reduce depression. There are hundreds of alternative strategies that could work for you.

Recap

Depression is a disorder that makes you feel less engaged in your own life, and it can make you unable to do ordinary tasks and enjoy things you usually enjoy. Depression robs you of joy, and it can disallow you to process your negative emotions as well, which can lead to further harm. Depression symptoms can include appetite changes, tiredness, moodiness, sadness, boredom, insomnia, rumination, and many others.

Depression can also be experienced in various ways and have a myriad of triggers. It can impact anyone, and no two cases of depression will look the same. Fortunately, depression is a treatable condition, but it is a serious condition that usually requires professional help from doctors and mental health professionals.

CHAPTER 5: THE WONDERS OF CBT

What is CBT?

Cognitive Behavioral Therapy (CBT) is an innovative and effective approach to psychotherapy that has helped millions of people worldwide manage and overcome a wide range of issues related to unwanted thoughts, feelings, and behaviors. One of CBT's most defining features is its focus on teaching people to be their own therapists. The idea is not to make you dependent on years of therapy but to teach you practical strategies and methods that you can use to deal with current problems right now and handle any future issues.

Depression, anxiety, and stress are some of the most common mental issues that people face every day, and CBT can provide you with solutions to these problems immediately. In this chapter, we will look at each of these in turn and outline strategies and methods you can use to take control of your mental health.

CBT is an evidence-based treatment that focuses on the relationship between thoughts, feelings, beliefs, and behaviors. It addresses dysfunctional emotions, destructive behaviors, and cognitive processes through several goal-oriented, systematic procedures. CBT is based on the cognitive model: how individuals perceive a situation is more meticulously connected to their reaction than the situation itself.

CBT can provide you with solutions to anxiety, stress, panic attacks, and depression, producing tangible results in a very short space of time. Most patients see progress in just a few months, but how long it takes for treatment to help depends on the individual. It can also depend on how often you seek treatment and how well you progress with your therapist (one therapist does not fit all). CBT treats a wide range of issues, so it is a cost-friendly and practical option for many people seeking psychological help. It is suitable for anyone who needs emotional support, not just persons with diagnosable conditions.

CBT is guided by a therapist or counselor who can bring awareness and instruct the patient on how to get better. It can be used on its own or in conjunction with other therapies. In some cases, it may be supplemented with medication, especially if someone's condition makes it hard for them to go to the CBT treatments or have the motivation to practice the skills learned in those sessions. It is often preferred because it is expedient and can more quickly get to the heart of issues.

CBT's primary goal is to show clients how they can recognize, challenge, and shift the cognitive patterns that have them stuck in a rut of repeating the same self-destructive behaviors based on their fears and other concerns. Unlike some other therapy methods, in CBT, your clinician serves as a guide who gives you skills, information, and instruction on how to practice and grow your awareness between sessions. Most of the work falls on you, and you have to put in time far beyond just the time you see your clinician.

CBT is an active process that calls upon the client to be fully engaged in their recovery process. You often have homework between sessions with CBT, and your clinician will instruct you to read specific works about your issue and log your behaviors and feelings between sessions. You will have to practice the skills your clinician teaches you in CBT repetitively so that they become habitual and become more comfortable for you to apply during difficult times. CBT will give you the coping skills and self-awareness that you need to improve your mental anguish, but it will take a considerable effort from you to make those changes. CBT is an excellent practice for people who are determined to get better, but it might be more challenging for people who are hesitant to challenge their cognitive patterns.

While CBT can often feel emotionally uncomfortable, CBT has few long-term risks. The risks that exist would mostly be caused by an ineffectual or immoral clinician, which is not usually the case. That's not to say that CBT won't cause you to cry, be angry, or address certain truths that you'd rather not address, but these hardships are hurdles you must get over if you want to get better. Sometimes, you must go through adversity to have victory, and that is often the case with CBT, but the practice is safe and highly renowned. However, if you have concerns, it is always a good idea to go over those concerns with your mental health professional during your first session.

Choosing a mental health professional that is right for you is an essential step in the process, and it is always good to do some research on clinicians in your area. You'll want to check their education and work experience, and you'll also want to note in what areas they specialize in. Finding someone who has the specialties that fit your needs is preferable when that option is available. Additionally, if the first person you see isn't a good fit, it is okay to look elsewhere. Therapy is a very individualized approach, and not all clinicians will fit with all clients.

Benefits of CBT

The abundance of benefits of CBT makes it a good choice for a wide range of issues. In CBT, the progress is mainly dependant on the patient, and a lot of the work occurs between sessions. The patient has accountability for their actions and treatment while the therapist is mostly a guide. This process allows CBT to be one of the fastest methods that you can choose. It can provide help while remaining cost-friendly to individuals and health care systems.

In some cases, CBT can work as well as medications. If you are wary of medications, CBT may be worth a shot, but it can also improve the outcomes started by medication and in conjunction with several other therapies. CBT is a flexible and convenient process, and those qualities appeal to most people.

CBT does a great job of connecting thoughts, emotions, and behaviors. It shows the profound connections between how we feel and how we act. As people go through life, they often begin to create flawed beliefs about the world and themselves. Therefore, these beliefs must be challenged with other beliefs that better reflect what people hope to accomplish. CBT highlights how mental processes contribute to your overall mental health, and by reorienting those processes rather than trying to defy them, you can resist anxiety, depression, and stress.

Some conditions may be too complex or severe for CBT alone, but CBT helps people understand themselves and learn how to change their situation by shifting their thought patterns. Plus, the skills you learn in CBT will help you in other areas of your life because this process gives you awareness of how your thoughts work, and it allows you to acknowledge how your emotions and thoughts can influence your feelings and behaviors. CBT has a wide range of benefits and little risk, which makes it all the more appealing. If you use CBT, you are sure to learn something, even if you don't fully cure your issues.

Core Beliefs

Your core beliefs are critical parts of CBT because these are the beliefs that shape your actions, and they are the integral beliefs that we have about who we are and the world. These beliefs tend to shift all our behaviors and emotional responses, which is why CBT makes them so central in its treatment. These beliefs are often assumptive, and we are prone to cognitive distortions and overgeneralizations. Your core beliefs can quickly become hazardous to your mental health (and even your physical health) if not addressed.

Examples of dangerous, common core beliefs:

- There's something inherently wrong about me

- I'll never be good enough

- No one will ever love me

- I am the worst employee in my division

- I am too fat to be cared for

- All the people are selfish

- I am a monster

- I give so much, but people give me so little

- People I love will abandon me

- I am weird

These are just some of the harmful core beliefs that many people have due to their pasts or societal standards, and if you have these beliefs or similar ones, they change the way you look at the world and the way you interact with others. Core beliefs are an integral part of CBT because they shape the experience you will have when you begin your work. When you start CBT, you will learn to spot negative core beliefs and begin to

114

eliminate them.

ABC Model

The ABC model is a standard CBT method that helps you acknowledge negative thought patterns. When you have cognitive distortions, this technique can help you question those thoughts. It follows the following framework:

A. Activating Event (the adversity that you face)

B. Beliefs (what you believe to be true about that event)

C. Consequences (the actions and emotions that resulted from the event)

In this model, the therapist assumes that B is a bridge connecting A and C; therefore, B is the subject you will focus most on. That fits the overall model of this therapy because CBT is focused on changing the core beliefs that cause you harm. When you have automatic thoughts as a response to activating events, you will start to recognize the beliefs you assume to be true, and you can then reshape those beliefs to create better outcomes.

As an example, if the person you are dating texts and cancels a date because they are sick (the activating event), you may have an automatic thought that *"They're lying. There's something wrong with me, and that's why they didn't show up"* (the belief). You may then start to feel sad, anxious, and ashamed (the consequences) because of the implication of that thought. You may even act irrationally and send a long, angry message to the other person, which only escalates the situation.

Your belief causes you unnecessary distress because your date very well could be telling you the truth, and your negative thoughts could create a rift in your relationship when your partner senses that you don't trust them. Thus, you can see how this same cycle (trigger, flawed belief, and response based on the flawed belief) can cause much tumult in a person's life unless the cycle is interrupted, which is what the ABC model does.

Practical Exercises

While it is best to seek help from a certified professional for CBT treatment, there are some common exercises that you can use to help with psychological issues. Knowing these methods can lead to immense personal growth. For persons tentative to get help, this information also helps you to know what to expect from CBT. These methods are all common ones used by professionals to teach their clients tools for combatting stress, depression, and anxiety.

Learning New Skills

Learning new skills can help clients address areas in which they are insufficient. These skills are taught in various ways that can include role play, models, and instructions. For people with stress, depression, or anxiety, skills can help them combat the negative thoughts and behaviors that contribute to their mental illness. Common skills include learning to express feelings and desires, problem-solving, confidence building, and interpersonal skills. The skills patients learn will depend on the nature of their problems and what skills they need most to combat their worries or mood imbalance.

Cognitive Restructuring

When you use cognitive restructuring, sometimes called cognitive reframing, you learn to study your negative thought patterns and pick them out. With this process, you can start to see when you tend to think in certain negative ways. For example, you may be prone to "Chicken Little syndrome," which is the idea that you jump to the worst conclusion when anything bad happens. You may also be prone to cognitive distortions, which cause you to over-generalize. As a result of these thought patterns, you become more distressed, and your anxiety, stress, and depression can worsen unless you address your cognitive processes. Once you are aware of your thought patterns, you can start to change them and shift the "sky is falling" attitude to an "I made a mistake, but it isn't the end of the world, and I know how to do better next time" attitude.

Activity Scheduling

For people with depression, an activity schedule is one CBT exercise that can help get them back into a more normal state. This method targets an activity that your depression may make it hard to complete, and it urges you to schedule time to do that task more often so that you can build up to that task becoming habitual. As you continue to do that task, you will feel rewarded, which will help your depression and allow you to do more. This exercise is one of the main parts of Behavioral Activation, which studies have found is one of the best ways to treat depression.

Guided Discovery

As one of the most helpful components of CBT, guided discovery is a method commonly used by clinicians. It is a process that helps clients uncover their mental processes so that they can later challenge them. Your anxiety, depression, or stress is caused because you have a fixed cognitive lens that you see the world through, but that lens is not always clear, and it can lead you to not be your best self. However, guided discovery challenges the responses that have become programmed into you, and it shows you how to see more clearly with new perceptions that are constructive rather than destructive.

Successive Approximation

In CBT, a successive approximation is a skill that allows people to take an overwhelming task and make it more approachable. This technique takes an overarching goal and breaks it down into increments to focus on one step at a time or ease themselves into a change. For instance, if you have an intense work task, it may seem impossible, but if you break that task into small subtasks, it becomes more manageable, and you don't feel as anxious about it.

Relaxation Training

Relaxation training is an excellent technique for people who feel stressed or anxious, and it is commonly used to help people who have high levels of worry that make it hard for them to keep a clear head. This technique is often used in addition to exposure techniques and cognitive restructuring. People who have high fear levels tend to have decreased reactivity in their parasympathetic nervous system, which is the section of the central nervous system that helps people calm down. This type of response usually occurs in "fight or flight" mode, in which your brain feels threatened and creates the physical response you have to stress or anxiety. Thus, relaxation training shows people how to get their parasympathetic nervous system to be less

121

lethargic. These techniques help people ease the physiological tension caused by anxiety to focus on the mental components that feed into that worry. Relaxation training uses a wide range of skills, including breathing skills and targeted muscle-relaxing skills.

Breathing Exercises

Taking charge of your breathing is one of the best ways to combat anxious feelings before they spiral out of control. Breathing techniques can be as simple as taking continuous deep breaths for five minutes; however, most clinicians will provide more detailed strategies.

A common breathing method used in CBT is called square breathing because it gets inhalations, exhalations, and pauses between breaths to be even, like the sides of a square. Be careful with this process if you have medical issues that are impacted by holding your breath, and stop if you start to feel like you have shallow breaths.

You begin this process by sitting in a quiet place for around fifteen minutes. It would help if you start by understanding how you usually breathe, and then you will want to expand the length of your baseline breath by one second to slow your breathing rate. Once you are used to the new rate, you can expand your breaths to be one second longer. Keep slowing down your breathing and stop when slowing it more would make it difficult to breathe. When your slow pace is established, you should begin to pause in equal lengths between inhaling and exhaling. Continue the process for about fifteen minutes.

Graded Exposure

Exposure is a technique that is used to help people address their fears. People learn to be less afraid of stimuli that cause anxiety by having repeated exposure to that thing. Mental health professionals will start slow and build up to introducing a person to what scares them. For example, suppose someone is afraid of a spider. In that case, they might start just by making a person watch a video of a spider, and eventually, they might have the fearful person touch the spider after several steps. Research has suggested that exposure therapy is one of the best techniques to help people reorient their cognitive patterns no matter their mental illness.

Mindfulness Meditation

Another popular CBT method is mindfulness meditation, which is used to overcome limiting thoughts and behavior patterns, to live healthier, happier, and more productive lives. Mindfulness will help you eliminate the effects of stress, clear and calm your mind, and experience freedom from emotional turmoil.

Mindfulness is the idea of learning how to be fully present and engaged in the moment, aware of your thoughts and feelings without distraction or judgment. It lays the foundation to build a stronger connection and relationship with yourself, allowing you to grow mentally and spiritually.

With mindfulness, people can stop fixating on certain fears or past occurrences, and they can learn to be present with their current feelings and situations.

CHAPTER 6: ROADBLOCKS TO OVERCOMING ANXIETY AND DEPRESSION

Common Obstacles

Several obstacles stand in the way of people not only recovering but staying in recovery. Even with treatment, negative behaviors can creep back into your life. Sadly, according to the Substance Abuse and Mental Health Services Administration, fifty-six percent of people who have mental illness in the United States do not have treatment for mental illness. This statistic highlights all the barriers that impede people from getting the help they need. No one likes living with stress, depression, or anxiety; nevertheless, millions of people worldwide suffer in silence, wondering if they'll ever have the happiness they crave.

Once someone accepts that they want to reach out for help, one of the most profound obstacles is the cost, and this cost impacts people on both an individual and societal level. Using data from MarketScan Databases, researchers have estimated that the average cost for treating an anxiety disorder is $6,475. For those suffering from a general anxiety disorder or panic disorder, the cost can increase by another thousand, or even two thousand. If a person has coexisting conditions, the price balloons even further. For example, if you have anxiety with comorbid depression, the price surges to nearly ten thousand dollars. The American Psychological Association estimates that depression is one of the most expensive health conditions in the United

States; it is the sixth most costly condition and costs Americans seventy-one billion each year. The need for treatment is large, and the costs of untreated issues only magnify the longer they go untreated

Another common obstacle that prevents people from getting help is a lack of awareness about these conditions. This lack of awareness can also make it challenging to facilitate a strong support system. Many people might not realize that there is something wrong with the way they are feeling. A major issue with the contributing thoughts of depression, anxiety, and stress is that they are all, to some degree, normal. Everyone feels down sometimes, just as everyone worries, so it's easy for people to think, "I am too emotional about this issue. I don't need help because it's not *that* bad." Further, your loved ones might not understand how your mental dysfunction impacts you, and they might make similarly dismissive comments. The continued raising of awareness of these issues is paramount.

Shame is another thing that blocks you from getting better, and this shame often stems from a lack of awareness. All the misconceptions about mental health results in internalized feelings of shame when you need mental help. Mental illnesses and mental health treatment carry stigmas. Even as people have an increased understanding of the importance of mental care, there's still a great deal of ignorance surrounding the topic. When you feel shame about something, you are more likely to keep it to yourself. Consequently, when you don't feel mentally healthy, you won't just avoid treatment, but you may even avoid turning to your support system because of that shame. For people with mental health issues, the guilt of those issues can deteriorate their condition and add undue stress to an already difficult situation.

The very nature of mental illnesses can make it

hard to improve. When people are depressed, they may not have the motivation to get treatment. Unfortunately, the nature of depression is that it commonly makes people feel unable to act. The acts required to get better can feel overtaxing and overwhelming. Likewise, Anxious people may let their anxiety prevent them from seeking the help they need. Common anxieties, like social anxiety, can feel like an impenetrable barrier between someone who needs help and the resources that can help them.

Similarly, stress can make you feel in over your head, and it makes you feel like you have too much to do in too little time. As a result, you may not think you have the time or energy to commit to treatment. In all these cases, the symptoms of your illness can make it a challenge to recover.

Too often, people give up on recovery when they have a bad day. People, especially those prone to perfectionism, commonly engage in all or nothing thinking. This type of thinking suggests that you can only win or lose, do wrong or right, be successful or fail. These core beliefs are falsehoods, but they can cause people trying to get better to think that treatment isn't working after just one bad day. Someone with social anxiety, for example, may build up their abilities through exposures, and they may be able to use coping skills to go to a big family reunion. The next week, though, they may go back to old ways and avoid a social event with their friends. In this case, they may start to have a negative thought that says, "I couldn't go out with my friends, so that must mean I am getting worse, not better." That thought likely doesn't reflect the truth. In recovery, you naturally have bad days, but if you were to look at the process in retrospect, you would see that the overall trend of your behaviors pointed towards progress.

Getting Unstuck

Remember that you have to work towards

recovering each day. Roadblocks will pop up periodically, but as long as you remain committed to doing better, you will have all the tools you need to problem-solve and overcome those roadblocks. When you have bad moments, use those moments to learn and improve your future decisions. You don't have to pressure yourself to be a perfect recovery machine. Take it at your own pace, and be merciful with yourself, especially when you have challenges.

If you have trouble affording services, there are other methods you can use, this book being one of them! Thousands of online resources can give you some insight into your condition and more detailed CBT exercises. You can also often find less expensive teletherapy options. Further, you can often find forums and support groups that are low cost or even free. These communities can make you feel less alone while helping you learn techniques that are commonly used in CBT and other therapies. Additionally, many professionals have financial options available to help you get treatment if you cannot otherwise get it through your healthcare. Your financial situation should never prevent you from getting help. There are plenty of avenues you can take that are inexpensive and will provide you with varying degrees of improvement.

Continue to research your condition so that you can increase your awareness. Learn as much as you can, and ask your doctors or mental health professionals questions when you have concerns. While it can feel uncomfortable to learn certain truths about ourselves, and it can be scary to realize how severe these conditions are, you cannot grow unless you allow those moments of discomfort to propel you forward. The more you dig, the more you will see that while anxiety, depression, and stress have serious impacts on your health and happiness, they are also highly treatable conditions. Armed with your knowledge, you can understand the hardships you will face on the road ahead.

Talk to your loved ones about your experiences. If they do not understand what you are going through, it usually isn't because they don't want to understand. Some people will indeed have biases that impede their understanding, but if there are people in your life who want to help you, don't keep them in the dark. Explain to them how your issues impact your overall well-being and get them involved with your recovery process. Update them when you feel better, and tell them if they do something that triggers you. You are entitled to a certain response from your loved ones, but being able to talk about your mental illness will help reduce the shame and stigma.

Don't let the shame stop you. While you cannot stop shame when it strikes, through treatment, you can learn to overcome the embarrassment and become more self-assured, so you don't have those same feelings next time. Learn the things that trigger your shame, and try to evaluate why you feel shame. Once you understand shame, you can handle the negative core beliefs that fuel that shame. Shame wants you to hide within yourself and have those negative core beliefs about who you are, but those feelings will only make your mental health worse. You can learn to resist those negative thought patterns.

It's up to you to choose what attitudes and core beliefs will lead to personal growth and happiness. While it is so much more complex than simply choosing to be mentally healthy versus remaining mentally ill (because we all want to be mentally healthy). That is fundamentally the choice you make every time you let destructive thoughts exist without acknowledgment. Mental illness often makes you feel out of control and disempowered, but you have the power to take steps forward, even if they are just small ones at first. Stop focusing on what you cannot control and look to the things you can control. When you do that, you'll form a whole new perspective, one that better meets your needs.

Accept that you can get better. Don't allow yourself to remain in the mindset that you are a "lost cause" because that's a cognitive distortion that changes the way you interact with the world, and that negativity will only make it harder to get better. You have to believe that there is something beyond your stress, depression, or anxiety because that belief will fuel you to push yourself. Remind yourself of the end goal because as distant as it may seem, it is waiting for you.

When you start to doubt yourself, remember yourself at five years old. Ask yourself, "What would I want for little me?" If you wouldn't want that sweet, innocent child to have to endure something, that means your adult self deserves better too. For example, if you have the repetitive thought, "I am the worst person alive," think of little you and imagine someone calling that young kid the worst person alive. When you use those words on a child, it feels inherently wrong because we naturally want to protect children. Children shouldn't feel like the worst people alive, and neither should you.

Fighting against stress, anxiety, and depression is often an uphill battle, which can be incredibly demoralizing for people who are already struggling. Recovery will sometimes feel awful, and it will be full of unexpected moments, some of them bad, some of them good. You'll have many victorious moments, and use those moments to give yourself momentum. Remember all the things you are fighting for. What is it that you want? Better focus? Improved relationships? A calmer existence? Whatever it is that pulls you forward, remember it when other factors threaten to pull you back.

Recap

No matter your situation, there are bound to be

obstacles that make it hard for you to recover from your issues. Perhaps, you struggle to accept that your problem is bad enough to get help. Maybe the finances don't work in your favor. You may feel ashamed of your mental health issues, or your support system might not be supportive. In many cases, the nature of your problem sways your thought patterns away from treatment. Even once you start the process, you may feel discouraged as ups and downs threaten your course. So much of recovery is creating awareness and learning that the obstacles are not the end of the world. When you address your negative core beliefs, you'll start to see that you're so much more resilient and capable than you think you are.

CHAPTER 7: ESTABLISHING A HAPPIER YOU

Shift Your Perspective

Renew your way of thinking. It helps to remember that thought patterns that were healthy at one point in your life can become stale and turn toxic. As you learn and have new needs and wants, you also have to learn to change your thinking. Just like you probably enjoy rearranging your house every so often, it's also nice to assess and refresh your thought patterns every so often. You're not the same person you were ten years ago, and you won't be the same person ten years from now, so what provides fulfillment now may fill you with dread in the future. Change is how you grow, so learn to move with it rather than trying to resist it.

Create a positive mindset. Be careful not to shift your negative thinking towards new negative ways of thinking. Finding positive outlooks to shape your worldview will help you resist mental conditions and stress. When negativity strikes, play devil's advocate and try to figure out how that negativity is false.

Break the pattern. The famous quote, *"If you want different results, you have to do things differently,"* is so profound. When you feel stuck or restless, all you have to do is to choose to act differently. What you're doing isn't working, so it cannot hurt to try acting in a way that you wouldn't normally. Challenge yourself to think in new ways.

Take action. Shifting your perspective is not just about how you think; it is also about what you do. While your thought patterns are the most influential factors when you use the CBT model, your behaviors are entangled with those thoughts, so the behaviors are not powerless. Changing your behaviors also changes your thoughts. As you start to act in new ways, your brain will get the memo and go along for the ride.

Start to affirm "I want to" rather than "have to." Otherwise, when you have to do something, it will feel like a chore. Wanting to do something is more enthusiastic, and it helps you choose options that reflect what you want to accomplish rather than what you feel pressured to complete.

If you have trouble breaking through the negativity, start with a small change in your view. For example, if you keep thinking, "I am worthless." Start to think about just one thing that

143

gives you worth, and say, "I do have worth." Then, whenever you catch yourself thinking that you are worthless, you can start to correct that thought process and build up to more fully recognizing ways that you do have worth. When things go wrong, find a silver lining.

Ask for the perspective of others. When you have trouble breaking from your limiting perspective, you can get feedback from other people because then you have more information that you can use to readjust your perspective. Considering other's views on a problem helps you see beyond your blind spots, and it teaches you that for every perspective you have, there is another one you can find.

Remain self-aware. Keep checking in with yourself to make sure your thought patterns aren't turning against you. When you lose awareness, that's when the stress, depression, and anxiety sneak into your life. New perspectives become old, so learn to identify when that is the case for you.

Focus on the New You

Self-Care and Relaxation

If you are working all the time and constantly running around, trying to get certain tasks done, you're going to be prone to stress and other mental dysfunctions, so you need to take care of yourself and find time for relaxation. Self-care is about calming down and investing time in yourself. It's doing anything that you feel you are lacking but would like to do.

Recognize that there's nothing wrong with needing to be alone sometimes, and you shouldn't feel guilty for treating yourself every once in a while either. It doesn't make you selfish to focus on yourself for a little time each day. You need that time to reorient your brain and recover from the daily stresses of your life.

Here are some tips to help with your journey:

- Make time for recreation. While many people neglect his need, you do need this time. During recreational times, you can do activities that you do simply because you love them.

- Have a spa day, so you can relax and escape the intensity of your life.

- Keep a journal to reflect on how you feel.

- If you are extroverted, spend extra time around other people and if you're introverted, take some spare time on your own during recreational hours.

- Stay in touch with your emotional and physical needs.

- Keep your treatment needs organized (using a calendar or other planning systems) to ensure you take medications and attend sessions or appointments that will keep you in top shape.

- Treat yourself to nice things every once in a while. It always feels rewarding to save up and have something special that we wouldn't usually get.

- Take time away from technology because technology can cause sleep problems, and it can distract you from your needs.

Appreciate the Great Outdoors

One of the greatest stress relievers is the great outdoors. The fresh air and the green wonders of the earth can revive your spirits. A whole branch of study called ecotherapy has emerged to study nature's precise role on people's well-being. When people spend more time in nature, they can reduce all three of the main mental health issues covered in this book.

The research is relatively new, so the exact reasons why nature is so beneficial is still not fully understood, but a 2015 study showed that the prefrontal cortex was more active when people walked in a natural environment rather than an urban one. The changes in the brain led to better mental health.

Additional research has uncovered that nature sounds also are good for your stress and anxiety levels. Natural sounds can cause a reduction of your blood pressure and cortisol, which is a hormone that spikes when you have a fight or flight response and feel stressed. Even if you cannot go outside, *Scientific Reports* created a 2017 report that showed that even recorded sounds of nature could have some of the same soothing effects. Additionally, merely seeing elements of nature has proven to calm people and distract them from their worries.

You don't need to spend a whole lot of time in

148

nature to start to see the effects. Any place in nature that you like will do. If you live in an urban area, finding a park or tending to houseplants or a community garden are suitable options. Even just half an hour per day can make you feel better, and you can combine getting your outdoor time with physical activity for extra stress-reduction.

Be Active!

Physical activity has long been a standard practice for overall health, but studies continue to show that it can be highly beneficial for your mental health as well. Exercise is known to increase feel-good hormones in your body, and research suggests that it creates more mental balance. Duke University completed a study that showed that people who didn't exercise were more likely to be depressed, and people who stopped exercising were more depressed than those who continued exercising or began to exercise. Therefore, exercise not only promotes mental health but it maintains it.

149

Researchers have also studied how exercise can prevent conditions such as diabetes, which has high depression rates. Mary de Groot says that people with diabetes (and other medical conditions) are more likely to become mentally ill, specifically depression. When they become mentally ill, their symptoms are more challenging to treat and more chronic than the general population. de Groot created a study in which she had depressed and diabetic patients begin to exercise. She found that CBT improved both their diabetes and their depression, showing how intertwined physical and mental conditions can be.

John Hopkins has corroborated the findings of other researchers who suggest that you also get a better night's sleep when you exercise more. Not only do people who regularly exercise sleep for longer, but they also get better quality sleep, and they fall asleep more quickly. Thus, exercise can help you feel happier and more well-rested.

Ensuring to get enough sleep is an essential part of feeling better.

Get Enough Sleep

When people get stressed or anxious, they often have trouble getting to sleep, or in some cases, they feel that they are too busy to sleep. In either case, sleep deprivation can have damaging consequences and worsen your mental health overall. People who have insomnia have an increased risk of depression, and in a pair of studies, the research showed that sleep problems often occurred before the depression. While in cases of anxiety, insomnia sometimes emerged before the anxiety, the connection wasn't as strong as it was with depression. While mental illness can worsen sleep problems, sleep problems can foreshadow mental illness.

Sleep complications are a common issue among the depressed, stressed, and anxious, and if you have this issue, it is essential to talk to your doctor to find tools you can use to get to sleep because it is hard to get better when you are sleep deprived. Exhaustion makes you think less clearly, and your ability to challenge your cognitive distortions will plummet.

Here are some common tips for a better night's sleep:

- Avoid looking at bright screens before bed (cellphone, television, etc.)

- Limit your caffeine and substance use

- Keep to a schedule to enforce your body's natural sleep cues

- Drink caffeine-free chamomile tea

- Ensure your room is dark when you sleep

- Use meditation and other relaxation skills

- Establish a bedtime routine

Feed Your Brain

Giving your brain certain nutrients can help you improve your attitude. According to Dr. Barish-Wreden, depression can improve by up to 60% with proper nutrition! With all the nutrients you need, your brain has the fuel it needs to have clarity and be more resilient to mental illness and stress. The American Dietetic Association says that eating habits are often impacted by mental illness, which then causes nutritional imbalances that make it even harder to improve your condition once you have it. Therefore, not only is a good diet a preventative measure, but it also impacts your ability to get better.

If your body doesn't have the nutrients it needs to run your vital systems, it starts to cut corners and become inefficient. Essential functions will be impaired and unable to run at optimal capacity.

An unbalanced diet makes you wearier and deficient in critical vitamins and minerals, which are both factors that can reduce your mental health outcomes. Additionally, nutritional imbalances can interfere with your hormone levels, which can trigger stress, depression, and anxiety.

Eating a balanced diet can make a profound change in your mental state, and a balanced diet starts with macronutrients— carbs, proteins, and fats. You'll want to include a balance of these foods in your diet unless your doctor tells you otherwise because they each play an essential role in your brain.

Our diet culture often conveys the idea that carbs are bad, and that's simply not the case. Your brain needs carbs to function. You should reach for complex carbs such as brown rice and other whole grains, rather than simple carbs like sugar or white bread. Whole grains do not eliminate nutritional parts of the grain in the processing process, so they have additional nutrients like fiber, which keep you balanced.

Fats are also a vital part of your diet. They are another type of food that people are taught is "bad." Fats help protect your organ, and they serve as energy stores between meals and keep you insulated. Nevertheless, some fats are more nutritionally dense than others. You will want to limit trans and unsaturated fats because they can harm your health. Some fats are vital, though. Omega-3 fatty acids, for example, found in fish like salmon, promote brain clarity, and omega-6 fatty acids, found in vegetable oils, are also known for improving mood conditions. Finally, monosaturated fats are healthy fats that can improve your overall health, and they can be found in sources like olive oil and avocados.

Proteins, found mostly in meat, eggs, dairy, and soy, are a building block for your body, and they allow you to repair tissues and build muscles. They have a varied and vital role in your body, and it's important to note that you'll want to eat these foods several times throughout the day because your body does not store them, so you use them as you eat them, which is why eating three meals a day is helpful.

Be careful of sugar. While there's not a problem with sugar in moderation, too much sugar can cause bodily inflammation. This inflammation can then result in depression and anxiety. Sugar is often something people reach for when they feel sad or stressed, so it can contribute to you struggling to have the nutritional balance you need to get better.

There are also herbal remedies. St. John's Wart is one that can help people who have milder depression, and multiple studies have suggested that it may be as impactful for mild depression as medications. Though, there are some things you should keep in mind with this herb before you take it. St. John's Wart may interfere with prescription medications that you take, and for people with anxiety, it can make you feel anxious in some cases. Thus, if you decide to take it, be sure to watch for symptoms and consult your doctor. Other herbs are known for their soothing qualities, and you can ingest them in teas or through aromatherapy. Chamomile and lavender are common choices. Herbal remedies likely won't cure your anxiety, but they can help as long as you are mindful of how you feel when you start these treatments.

Several vitamin deficiencies also result in worsened mental health. Vitamin B-12 and vitamin B-6 are also good nutritional choices because these vitamins partake in the production and use of chemicals in your brain that control mood. As a result, low levels can result in depression or a lower mood. Not much research has shown conclusively that these vitamins are a suitable treatment for depression, but they contribute to a worsened condition if you are deficient. Vitamin D is another essential vitamin that many people are lacking. You get this vitamin through supplement or sunlight, so you might not have enough when you guard your skin from the sun or in the winter months. A 2013 meta-analysis showed that people who had low vitamin D also had significantly higher risks of depression. Ensuring you have all the vitamins and nutrients you need is one step you can take to improve your symptoms and resist the formation of new symptoms.

Visualization, Meditation, and Mindfulness

Visualization is a skill that helps people envision a brighter future. When you visualize, you use imagery to create a mental picture of what you want to achieve. For example, you could imagine your anxiety as a heavy weight that pins you to the floor, and you could imagine your treatment as the strength you need to free yourself of that weight. By imagining in such a visceral way, your brain clings to the messages you are trying to promote. As you continue to use this practice, you can reshape your mental processes.

Visualization is often linked to new age spiritual practice, but neuroscientific and psychological research backs it up. One prominent study in the *Frontiers in Human Neuroscience* journal shows that this practice can positively change how the brain is wired. In other studies, people who practiced self-guided visualization had fewer depression symptoms and better mental health. The research suggested that one neurotransmitter associated with lower stress and worry, GABA, became more prominent in those who visualized. While visualization is future-thinking, it does so positively, rather than in a way that promotes negative thinking.

Visualization helps you to envision a better future;

159

however, meditation and mindfulness help you focus on what you can do right now to create that better future. These practices are about processing what you are feeling without judgment or obsession. They are now-oriented rather than becoming fixated on the fears caused by the past or the worries of the future. Mindfulness meditation, as you've learned, is a common technique in CBT. Various studies have supported this method, and evidence suggests that this practice makes your pre-frontal cortex more active, which is the part of your brain that makes you feel positive emotions. Mediation is just one common process of being mindful, and it helps you be aware of your connection with yourself. You can apply mindfulness to all areas of your life— food, exercise, work— because when you are mindful about your behaviors, you can understand how they make you feel as you do them, which allows you to then behave in ways that make you feel better.

Have a Support System

A support system is a vital part of your mental health. One 2015 survey showed that people with a support system willing to help them emotionally had a decreased average stress level. A support system gives you people who will listen to your problems and allow you to express your emotional state. It prevents social isolation, which is a known factor that makes people more at risk for mental illness. Mental Health First Aid suggests that a sound support system has anywhere from one to ten people representing various parts of your life (work, family, hobbies, etc.). Your support system will take time for you to create because trust takes time, so take that time to build it well and ensure you choose people who will unselfishly support you and call you out when needed.

<u>Recap</u>

To establish a happier you, you need to start by shifting your perspective to a healthier one, and you can do this by being aware of your current perspective and addressing how that perspective helps you rather than harms you. You need to actively work towards changing your view because if you don't put in diligent work, nothing will ever change. Beyond just shifting your perspective, which can take extensive work, there are simple steps you can take to improve your mental state. These are things you can start right now without any professional help. For many, these things may seem basic, but you forget how important they are when your head is foggy from mental illness or stress.

The first thing you can do is establish a routine of self-care and relaxation, which is a way of appreciating yourself. A stroll outside or standing in the fresh air can renew your spirits, just as sleep can restore your body. Additionally, remaining active and keeping a healthy diet ensures your body is healthy. When your body is healthy, it is more resilient to distress, and you have the energy you need to fight any issues you have. Tools like daily visualization, meditation, and mindfulness can help you be more present and take charge of the things you can control rather than focusing on what you can't. Finally, establishing a support system can give you a team that will pick you up when hardships make you want to stay down.

CONCLUSION

Being overwhelmed with certain aspects of your life is normal, especially in the fast-paced, hyperactive society we live in. The pressure of balancing work or academic expectations and personal life can be challenging. With all of life's ups and downs, coping with stress is problematic and can result in you losing your vibrancy. Without treatment, the resulting negative feelings and thought patterns can worsen and become chronic, leaving you wondering if you'll ever accomplish your dreams and goals. You may feel like an outsider due to your issues, but you're not weird or strange. You are part of a group of millions of people who are overwhelmed just like you.

Mental health issues result from how the brain inherently functions. The human brain finds patterns, and based on past experiences, reacts accordingly. Ingrained negative thoughts can be hard to overcome. Cognitive distortions can fuel the misperception of certain situations, making it hard to see beyond the generalizations and assumptions. Once you become aware of your misperceptions, only then can you start to change them.

With stress levels being at an all-time high worldwide, mental illness can impact virtually everyone on earth at some point. It is vital to find the source of your mental unhappiness, as this will illuminate the changes you should make. Whether you have mild issues or severe issues, putting a name to what you are feeling can help you get on the right recovery path and understand what you are up against. Try to seek help as soon as you can because the longer issues linger, the more entrenched negative core beliefs become, and the harder they will be to break.

The Anxiety and Depression Association of America suggests that only around 37 percent of people suffering from anxiety receive treatment, despite these conditions being treatable. It means that a large portion of anxiety-sufferers are living with their conditions unnecessarily. If you have anxiety, you may feel on edge and moody because fear sets off reactions in your brain, and you may also experience physical symptoms of anxiety, which can be draining. Anxiety interferes with your social life and relationships – which may suffer as your behavior becomes self-sabotaging. When it lingers, anxiety can become a paralyzing force, commonly making it harder to get your work done and increasing the odds of physical and additional mental conditions.

According to the World Health Organization, depression is the fourth leading cause of disability globally, meaning it carries a high societal cost beyond treatment costs. Depression can strike when you have a traumatic life event, or you may simply be prone to a depressed mood. Either way, it can stop you from feeling fully engaged in your life. When depressed, you have trouble truly embracing your feelings, making it hard to feel any joy. Depression can be experienced in a myriad of ways and different degrees, but no matter the type of depression, learning coping mechanisms allows you to get back to enjoying the things you love and experience the world with more vigor.

Stress is the most prevalent of all the issues discussed in this book because it is common among all people. It is estimated that stress costs the country 300 billion dollars every year in the

United States alone. People's stress accumulates quickly over time, lessening their productivity, health, and overall ability to lead high-quality lives. Many factors can cause stress, and the most common seem to occur in the workplace. Work assignments, colleagues, and the pressure to succeed can make for a stressful day. Because most people have to work, new ways and new skills must be found to help you breathe through your stress, allowing you to resist it when it starts creeping up on you.

One of the most transformative ways to address negative thought patterns is cognitive-behavioral therapy. In a meta-analysis of over two hundred studies, Hofmann et al. found that CBT had comparable results to medicative treatment for chronic depression and promising results compared to no treatment at all. Some researchers found that CBT patients had better results at a six-month check-in; additionally, they found that CBT was an excellent first approach to anxiety because it provided long-term improvement skills. CBT is a well-studied therapy that many patients use to take charge of their recovery and learn how to rewire their thought patterns to reinforce more positive ideas. One of CBT's best aspects is that lasting changes are created within months of treatment; it teaches you to apply new skills and cope with the challenges that usually would have caused negative responses. This treatment can work independently or in conjunction with other mental health efforts to customize the experience based on your needs.

You can learn to become a new and happier you using the tools and techniques provided in this book. With simple self-care methods, professional treatment, and newfound attention to your mental well-being and thought patterns, your awareness will lead you to new opportunities that you had never considered. Negative beliefs cause self-limitation, but by bringing those beliefs to the fore, you begin to confront the limitations. While

170

some of these habits are basic, gradual steps forward add up and create immense changes over time.

There will be challenges as you seek recovery; however, there is light at the end of the tunnel. When you put in the effort and allow yourself to have hope, you've already started to shift the mindset that confounds you. As you embark on your journey, you may cry, and you may feel upset, but those feelings are all a part of the process because recovery requires you to face some uncomfortable truths. You cannot allow that discomfort to discourage you from persevering.

Your depression, anxiety, or stress should not keep you from living your life to the fullest. It's time to tear down your current way of thinking and rebuild thought patterns that contribute to your life in constructive ways.

One more thing

If you enjoyed this book and found it helpful, I'd be very grateful if you'd post a short review on Amazon. Your support does make a difference, and I read all the reviews personally so I can get your feedback and make this book even better. I love hearing from my readers, and I'd really appreciate it if you leave your honest feedback.

Thank you for reading!

Also by Richard Banks

How to Stop Being Negative, Angry, and Mean:
Master Your Mind and Take Control of Your Life

How to Deal with Grief, Loss, and Death: A Survivor's
Guide to Coping with Pain and Trauma, and Learning
to Live Again

Develop a Positive Mindset and Attract the Life of
Your Dreams: Unleash Positive Thinking to Achieve
Unbound Happiness, Health, and Success

The Keys to Being Brilliantly Confident and More
Assertive: A Vital Guide to Enhancing Your
Communication Skills, Getting Rid of Anxiety, and
Building Assertiveness

How to be Charismatic, Develop Confidence, and
Exude Leadership: The Miracle Formula for Magnetic
Charisma, Defeating Anxiety, and Winning at
Communication

REFERENCES

Ackerman, C. E. (2020, October 31). *Cognitive Distortions: When Your Brain Lies to You (+ PDF Worksheets)*. PositivePsychology.Com. https://positivepsychology.com/cognitive-distortions/

Alternative Therapies for Depression. (n.d.). Cleveland Clinic. Retrieved December 18, 2020, from https://my.clevelandclinic.org/health/treatments/9303-depression-alternative-therapies

American Psychological Association. (2018, October 28). *What's the Difference Between Stress and Anxiety*. https://www.apa.org/topics/stress-anxiety-difference

Anxiety and Depression Association of America. (n.d.). *Therapy Options*. Retrieved December

17, 2020, from https://adaa.org/finding-help/treatment/therapy

Barish-Wreden, M. (n.d.). *Eating Well for Mental Health | Sutter Health*. Sitter Health. Retrieved December 18, 2020, from https://www.sutterhealth.org/health/nutrition/eating-well-for-mental-health

Bauer, B. A. (2018, March 2). *Herbal treatment for anxiety: Is it effective?* Mayo Clinic. https://www.mayoclinic.org/diseases-conditions/generalized-anxiety-disorder/expert-answers/herbal-treatment-for-anxiety/faq-20057945

Batz, C. (2019, October 2). *How Trauma Changes the Brain*. The Independence Center. https://www.theindependencecenter.org/how-trauma-changes-the-brain/

Borchard, T. (2017, November 15). *14 Instant Ways to*

Calm Yourself Down | Everyday Health. EverydayHealth.Com. https://www.everydayhealth.com/columns/ther ese-borchard-sanity-break/10-quick-ways-to-calm-down/

Bonfil, A. (2013, August 18). *Reduce Anxiety Quickly with Square Breathing*. Cognitive Behavioral Therapy Los Angeles. https://cogbtherapy.com/cbt-blog/2013/08/reduce-anxiety-quickly-with-square.html

Boyd, D. (2019, December 18). *Daily Life*. The American Institute of Stress. https://www.stress.org/daily-life

Boyle, M. A. (2015). *Personal Nutrition* (9th ed.). Cengage Learning.

Bremner, D. J. (2006). *Traumatic stress: effects on the brain*. PubMed.

https://pubmed.ncbi.nlm.nih.gov/17290802/

Bruce, D. F. (2008a, May 21). *Psychotic Depression.* WebMD. https://www.webmd.com/depression/guide/psychotic-depression#1

Bruce, D. F. (2008b, May 22). *Types of Depression.* WebMD. https://www.webmd.com/depression/guide/depression-types#3

Canadian Mental Health Association. (n.d.). *Connection Between Mental and Physical Health.* Retrieved December 2, 2020, from https://ontario.cmha.ca/documents/connection-between-mental-and-physical-health/

Canadian Mental Health Association. (n.d.). *The Relationship between Mental Health, Mental Illness and Chronic Physical Conditions.*

Retrieved December 9, 2020, from https://ontario.cmha.ca/documents/the-relationship-between-mental-health-mental-illness-and-chronic-physical-conditions/

Center, C. W. (2019, June 29). *What Prevents People from Seeking Mental Health Treatment?* Clearview Women's Center | BPD Treatment Los Angeles. https://www.clearviewwomenscenter.com/blog/mental-health-treatment-obstacles/

Cognitive behavioral therapy - Mayo Clinic. (2019, March 16). Mayo Clinic. https://www.mayoclinic.org/tests-procedures/cognitive-behavioral-therapy/about/pac-20384610

Cognitive Behavioral Therapy Exercises. (n.d.). Cognitive Behavioral Therapy Los Angeles. Retrieved December 17, 2020, from https://cogbtherapy.com/cognitive-behavioral-therapy-exercises

Cognitive Behavioral Therapy Los Angeles. (n.d.). *Relaxation Training using CBT Los Angeles | CBT Relaxation Therapy*. Retrieved December 17, 2020, from https://cogbtherapy.com/relaxation-training-los-angeles

Cuncic, A. (2020, March 20). *Things to Start Doing If You Have Social Anxiety Disorder*. Verywell Mind. https://www.verywellmind.com/social-anxiety-disorder-tips-3024209

Dekin, S. (2019, July 29). *How Does Self-Care Affect Mental Health?* Mission Harbor Behavioral Health. https://sbtreatment.com/blog/self-care-affect-mental-health/

Dingfelder, S. F. (2009, August). *Stigma: Alive and Well*. American Psychological Association. https://www.apa.org/monitor/2009/06/stigma

Facts & Statistics | Anxiety and Depression Association of America, ADAA. (n.d.). Anxiety and Depression Association of America. Retrieved December 2, 2020, from https://adaa.org/about-adaa/press-room/facts-statistics

Gabbey, A. E. (2018, September 3). *Persistent Depressive Disorder (Dysthymia)*. Healthline. https://www.healthline.com/health/dysthymia

Felman, A. (2020, January 11). *What to know about anxiety*. Medical News Today. https://www.medicalnewstoday.com/articles/323454

Exercising for Better Sleep. (n.d.). Johns Hopkins Medicine. https://www.hopkinsmedicine.org/health/wellness-and-prevention/exercising-for-better-sleep

Global Organization for Stress. (2018, December 12). *STRESS   FACTS*. http://www.gostress.com/stress-facts/

Hall-Flavin, D. K. (2018, June 1). *Vitamin B-12 and depression: Are they related?* Mayo Clinic. https://www.mayoclinic.org/diseases-conditions/depression/expert-answers/vitamin-b12-and-depression/faq-20058077

Harvard Health Publishing. (2019, February). *Past trauma may haunt your future health*. Harvard Health. https://www.health.harvard.edu/diseases-and-conditions/past-trauma-may-haunt-your-future-health

Harvard Health Publishing. (n.d.). *Sour mood getting you down? Get back to nature*. Harvard Health. https://www.health.harvard.edu/mind-and-mood/sour-mood-getting-you-down-get-back-to-nature

Harvard Health Publishing. (2019, March 18). *Sleep and mental health*. Harvard Health. https://www.health.harvard.edu/newsletter_art icle/sleep-and-mental-health

Healthline Editorial Team. (2020, February 25). *Everything You Need to Know About Stress*. Healthline. https://www.healthline.com/health/stress#type s

Higuera, V. (2020, February 11). *Everything You Want to Know About Depression*. Healthline. https://www.healthline.com/health/depression

Hofmann, S. G., Asnaani, A., Vonk, I. J. J., Sawyer, A. T., & Fang, A. (2012, July 31). *The Efficacy of Cognitive Behavioral Therapy: A Review of Meta-analyses*. Cognitive Therapy and Research. https://link.springer.com/article/10.1007/s1060 8-012-9476-

1?error=cookies_not_supported&code=2e6d0
934-45ca-4959-8135-18149db6abbd

Holland, K. (2018, August 20). *Cognitive-Behavioral Therapy for Depression.* Healthline. https://www.healthline.com/health/depression/cognitive-behavioral-therapy

How Beliefs Are Formed and How to Change Them. (n.d.). Skilled at Life. Retrieved December 9, 2020, from http://www.skilledatlife.com/how-beliefs-are-formed-and-how-to-change-them/

Hull, M. (2020, September 30). *Mental Health Statistics.* The Recovery Village Drug and Alcohol Rehab. https://www.therecoveryvillage.com/mental-health/related/mental-illness-statistics/

Jennings, K. A. (2018, August 28). *16 Ways to Relieve Stress.* Healthline. https://www.healthline.com/nutrition/16-ways-relieve-stress-anxiety

Kapil, R. (2020, August 6). *The Importance of Having a Support System*. Mental Health First Aid. https://www.mentalhealthfirstaid.org/2020/08/the-importance-of-having-a-support-system/

LeBlanc, N. J., & Marques, L. (2019, April 15). *How to handle stress at work*. Harvard Health Blog. https://www.health.harvard.edu/blog/how-to-handle-stress-at-work-2019041716436

Legg, T. J. (2020, April 17). *What is the ABC Model of Cognitive Behavioral Therapy?* Healthline. https://www.healthline.com/health/abc-model#how-it-works

Less Wrong. (n.d.). *The Map Is Not The Territory*. Retrieved December 9, 2020, from https://www.lesswrong.com/tag/the-map-is-not-the-territory

Massachusetts Institute of Technology. (2012, May 17). *Are Habits More Powerful Than Decisions? Marketers Hope So.* MIT Sloan Management Review. https://sloanreview.mit.edu/article/are-habits-more-powerful-than-decisions-marketers-hope-so/

Mayo Clinic Staff. (2017, October 13). *St. John's wort*. Mayo Clinic. https://www.mayoclinic.org/drugs-supplements-st-johns-wort/art-20362212

Mental Health America. (n.d.). *Quick Facts and Statistics About Mental Health*. Retrieved December 2, 2020, from https://www.mhanational.org/mentalhealthfacts

Mental Health Foundation. (2020, February 20). *Mindfulness*. https://www.mentalhealth.org.uk/a-to-z/m/mindfulness

Mental Health Foundation. (2020, February 10). *Physical health and mental health.* https://www.mentalhealth.org.uk/a-to-z/p/physical-health-and-mental-health‘

Mohney, G. (2018, January 15). *Stress Costs U.S. $300 Billion Every Year.* Healthline. https://www.healthline.com/health-news/stress-health-costs#How-stress-impacts-certain-groups-

NHS website. (2020, November 13). *10 stress busters.* Nhs.Uk. https://www.nhs.uk/conditions/stress-anxiety-depression/reduce-stress/

Overcoming Barriers to Treatment. (2018, October 8). Pasadena Villa. https://www.pasadenavilla.com/2018/10/08/overcoming-barriers-to-treatment/

Pros & Cons of CBT Therapy | The CBT Therapy Clinic – Nottingham – West Bridgford. (n.d.). The CBT Clinic. Retrieved December 18, 2020, from http://www.thecbtclinic.com/pros-cons-of-cbt-therapy

Raypole, C. (2018, October 10). *6 Pressure Points for Anxiety Relief.* Healthline. https://www.healthline.com/health/pressure-points-for-anxiety

Riopel, L. M. (2020, September 1). *8 Benefits of Cognitive Behavioral Therapy (CBT) According to Science.* PositivePsychology.Com. https://positivepsychology.com/benefits-of-cbt/

Ritchie, H. (2018, January 20). *Mental Health.* Our World in Data. Retrieved December 2, 2020, from https://ourworldindata.org/mental-health

Rizzo, S. (2016, April 20). *Your Thoughts Create Your Beliefs.* SUCCESS. https://www.success.com/your-thoughts-create-your-beliefs/

Russel, D. (2018, October 31). *Overcoming Barriers to Recovery | NAMI: National Alliance on Mental Illness.* National Alliance on Mental Illness. https://www.nami.org/Blogs/NAMI-Blog/October-2018/Overcoming-Barriers-to-Recovery

Scaccia, A. (2020, August 26). *Is a Vitamin D Deficiency Causing Your Depression?* Healthline. https://www.healthline.com/health/depression-and-vitamin-d

Schimelpfening, N. (2020, December 9). *Does Depression Go Away on Its Own With Time?* Verywell Mind. https://www.verywellmind.com/can-depression-stop-without-treatment-1067582

Scott, E. (2020, January 8). *17 Highly Effective Stress Relievers.* Verywell Mind. https://www.verywellmind.com/tips-to-reduce-stress-3145195

Scott, E. (2020, June 29). *What Are the Main Causes of Stress?* Verywell Mind. https://www.verywellmind.com/what-are-the-main-causes-of-stress-3145063

Spannhake, J. (2020, November 20). *Five Ways to Shift Your Perspective.* Attorney at Work. https://www.attorneyatwork.com/5-ways-shift-perspective/

Star, K. (2020, April 10). *How Thoughts and Values May Affect Your Anxiety.* Verywell Mind. https://www.verywellmind.com/negative-thinking-patterns-and-beliefs-2584084

Star, K. (2020, September 30). *Visualization Techniques Can Help Manage Your Symptoms.* Verywell Mind. https://www.verywellmind.com/visualization-for-relaxation-2584112

Sweeton, J. (2017, February 23). *Here's Your Brain on Trauma.* Dr. Jennifer Sweeton. https://www.jennifersweeton.com/blog/2017/3/14/heres-your-brain-on-trauma

Therapy, H. (2019, October 19). *Core Beliefs in CBT – Identifying And Analysing Your Personal Beliefs.* Harley Therapy™ Blog. https://www.harleytherapy.co.uk/counselling/core-beliefs-cbt.htm

The National Council for Behavioral Health. (n.d.). *Trauma Infographic.* Retrieved December 9, 2020, from https://www.thenationalcouncil.org/wp-content/uploads/2013/05/Trauma-infographic.pdf?daf=375ateTbd56

The Power of Positive Thinking. (n.d.). Johns Hopkins Medicine. Retrieved December 2, 2020, from https://www.hopkinsmedicine.org/health/welln ess-and-prevention/the-power-of-positive-thinking?amp=true

Villines, Z. (2017, March 23). *Visualization Can Improve Mood, Support Mental Health*. GoodTherapy.Org Therapy Blog. https://www.goodtherapy.org/blog/visualizatio n-can-improve-mood-support-mental-health-0323171

What Happens When You Have a Panic Attack. (2019). WebMD. https://www.webmd.com/anxiety-panic/ss/slideshow-panic-attack

What does "suicide contagion" mean, and what can be done to prevent it. (2019, February 25). HHS.Gov.